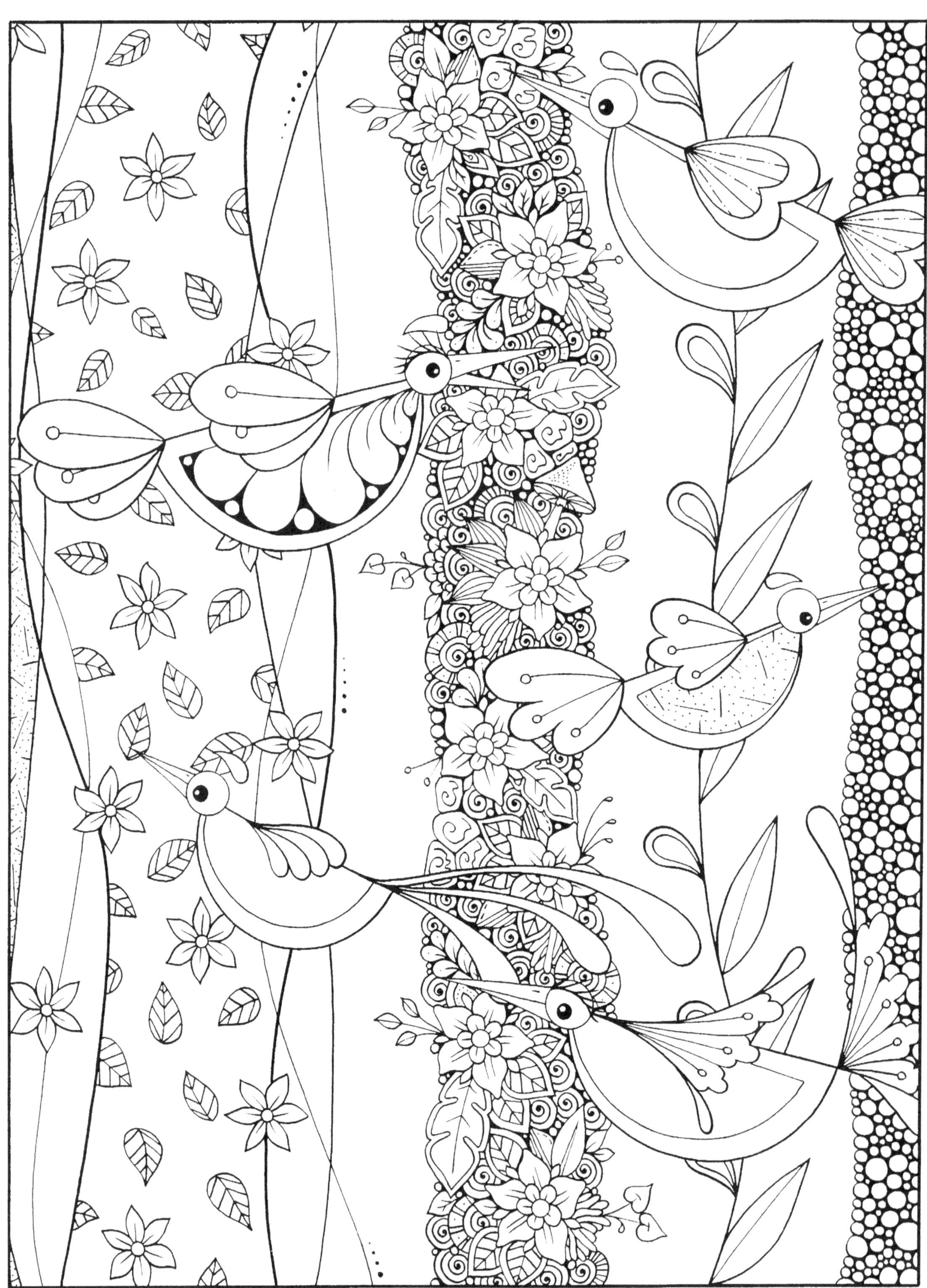

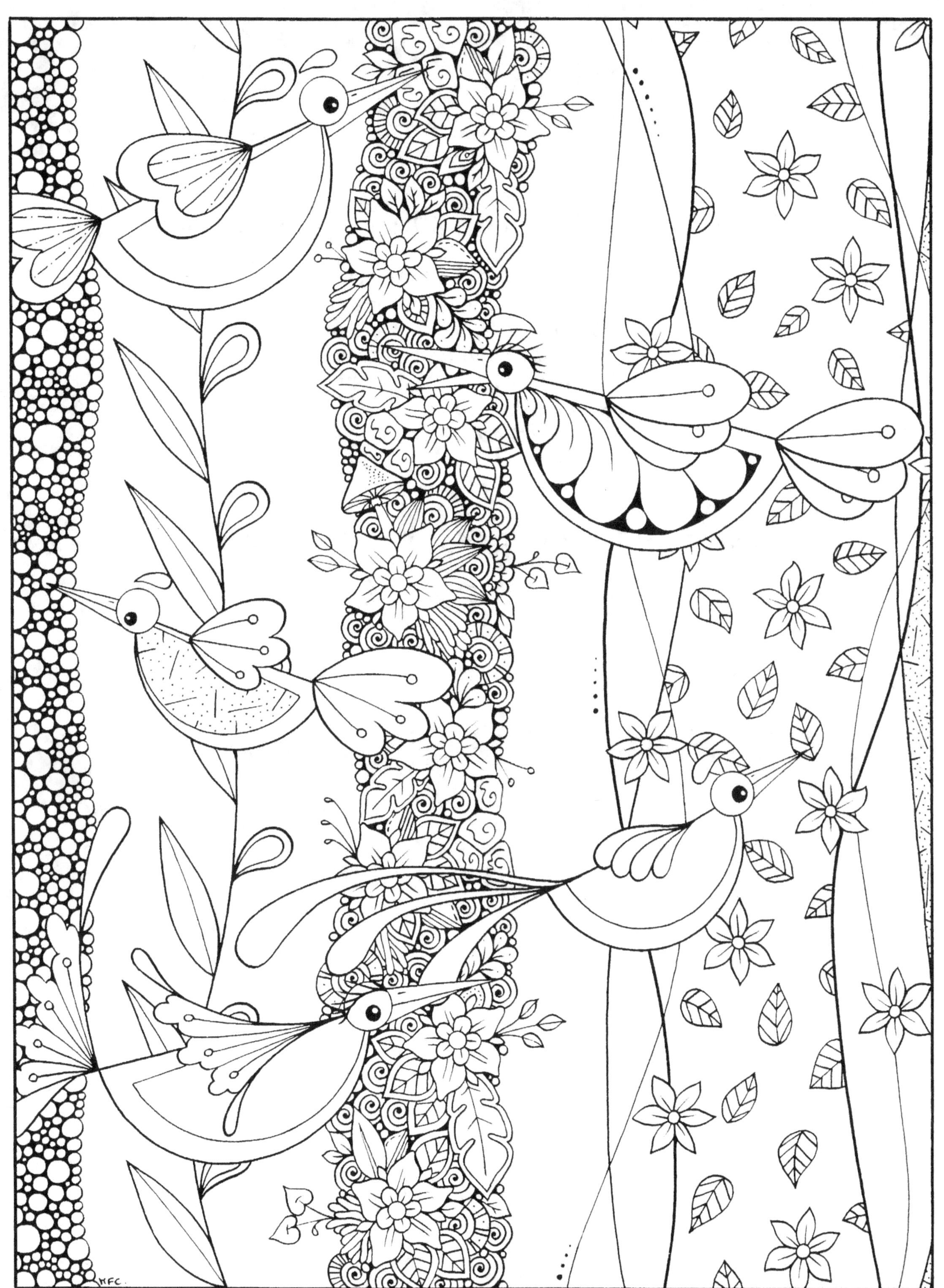

Coloring books available on Amazon :

- The feet in the water
- A pencil on the Heart
- Color your Kimmidoll
- Back to the sea
- MFC Doodle's Book
- Enchanted Menagerie
- Walk in Seasons

Book published by Blue Star Coloring

- Color Couture

Welcome to Birdsland

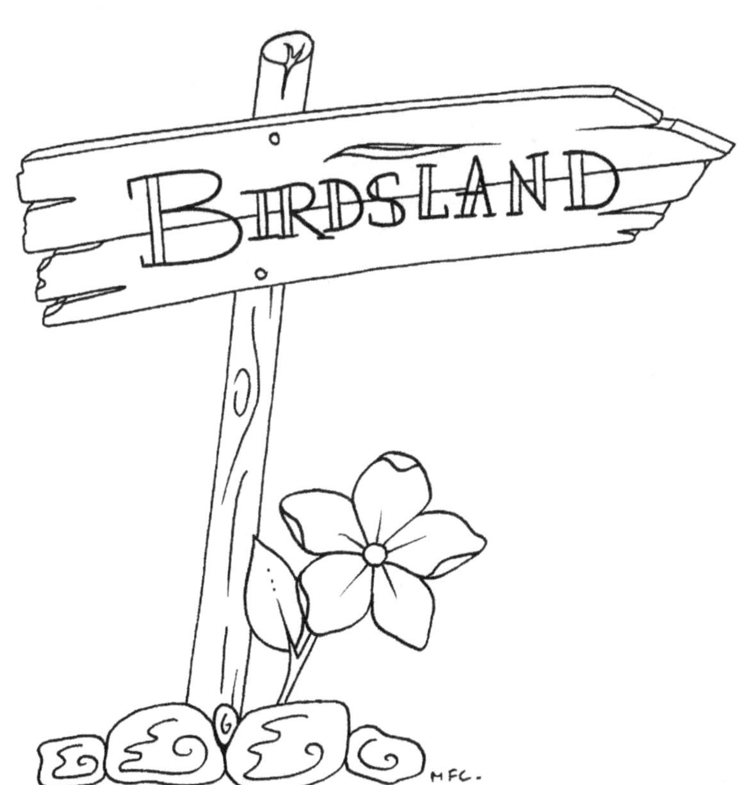

Maud Feral-Chauveau

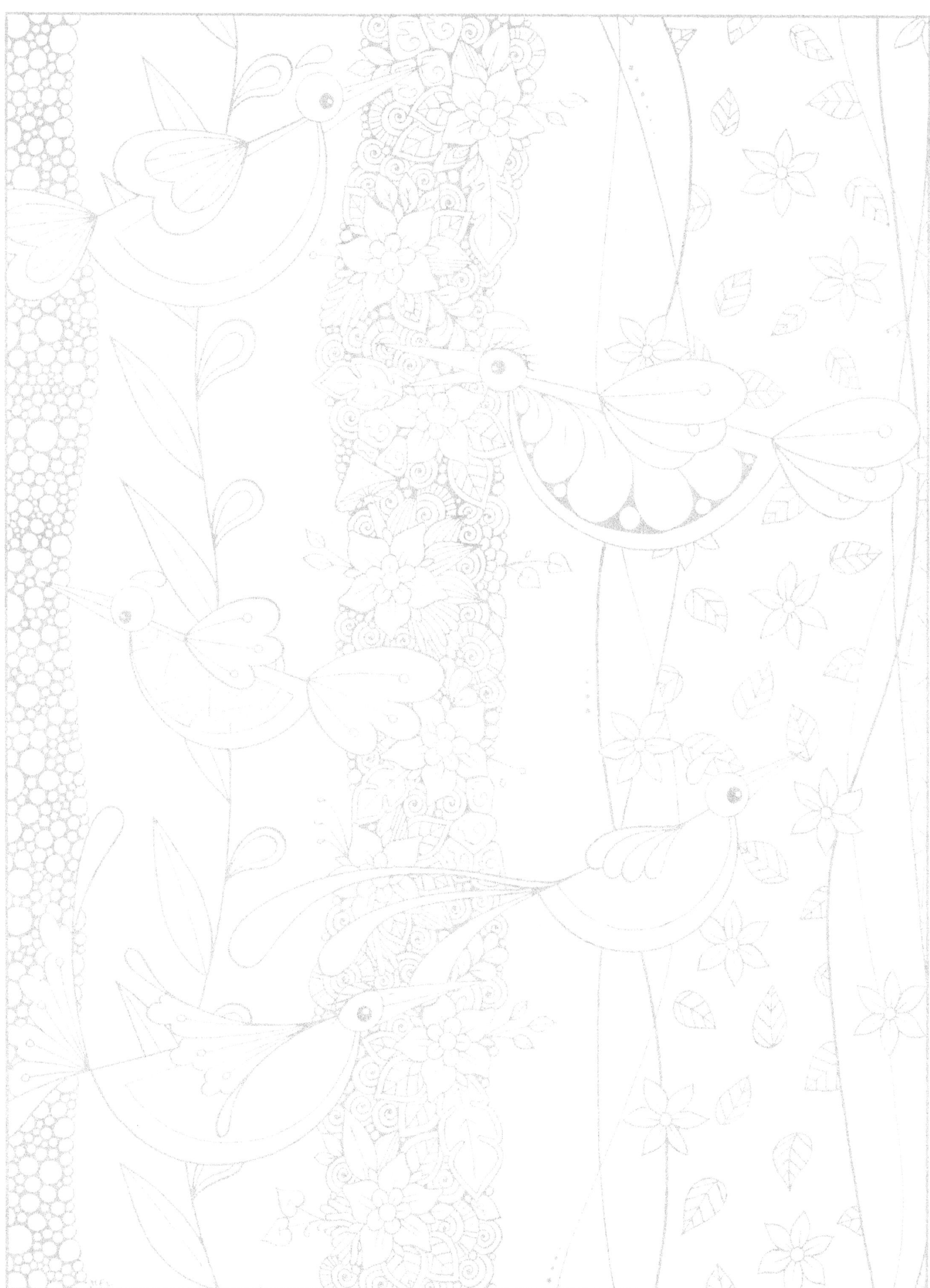

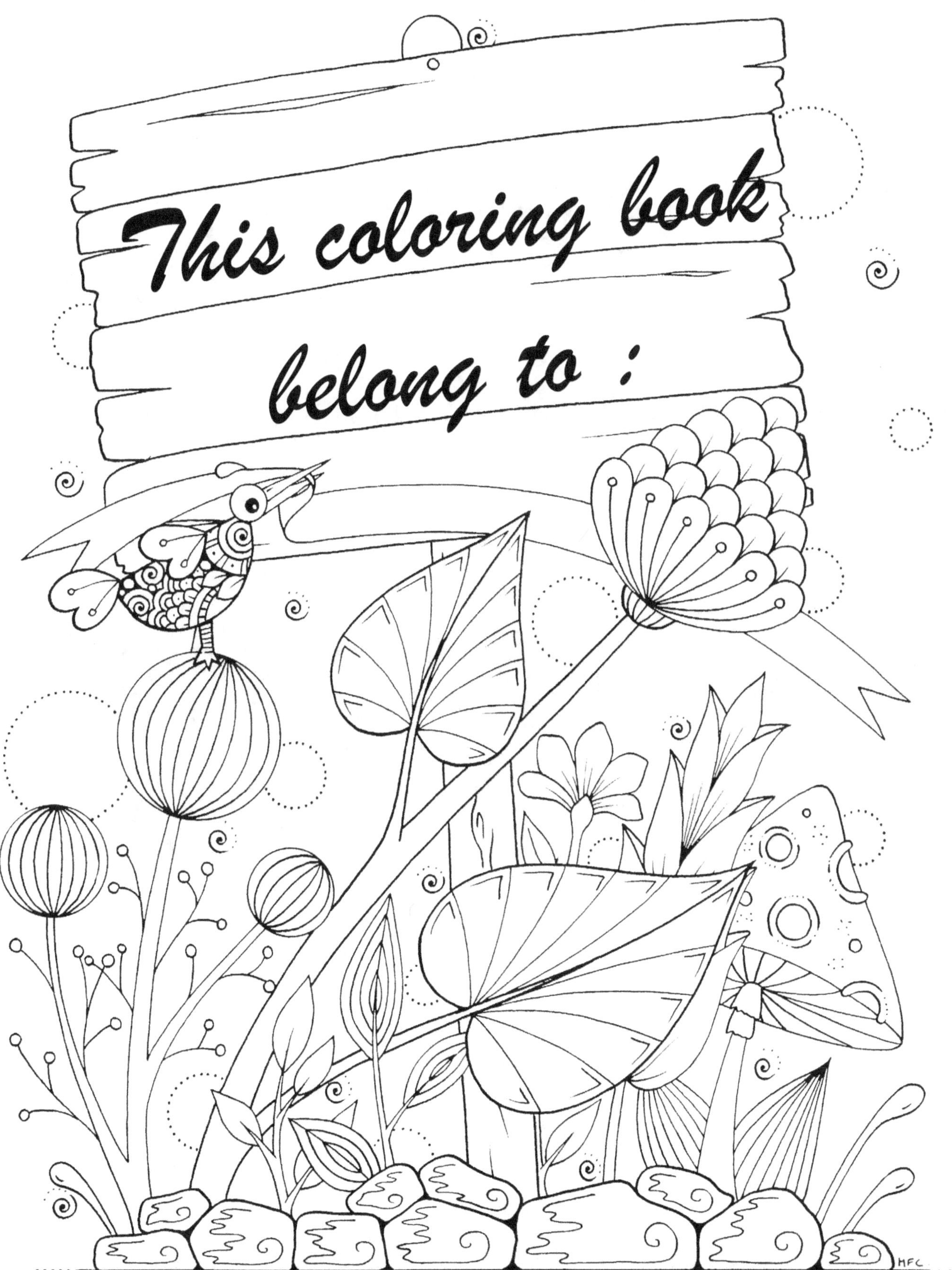

This coloring book
belong to :

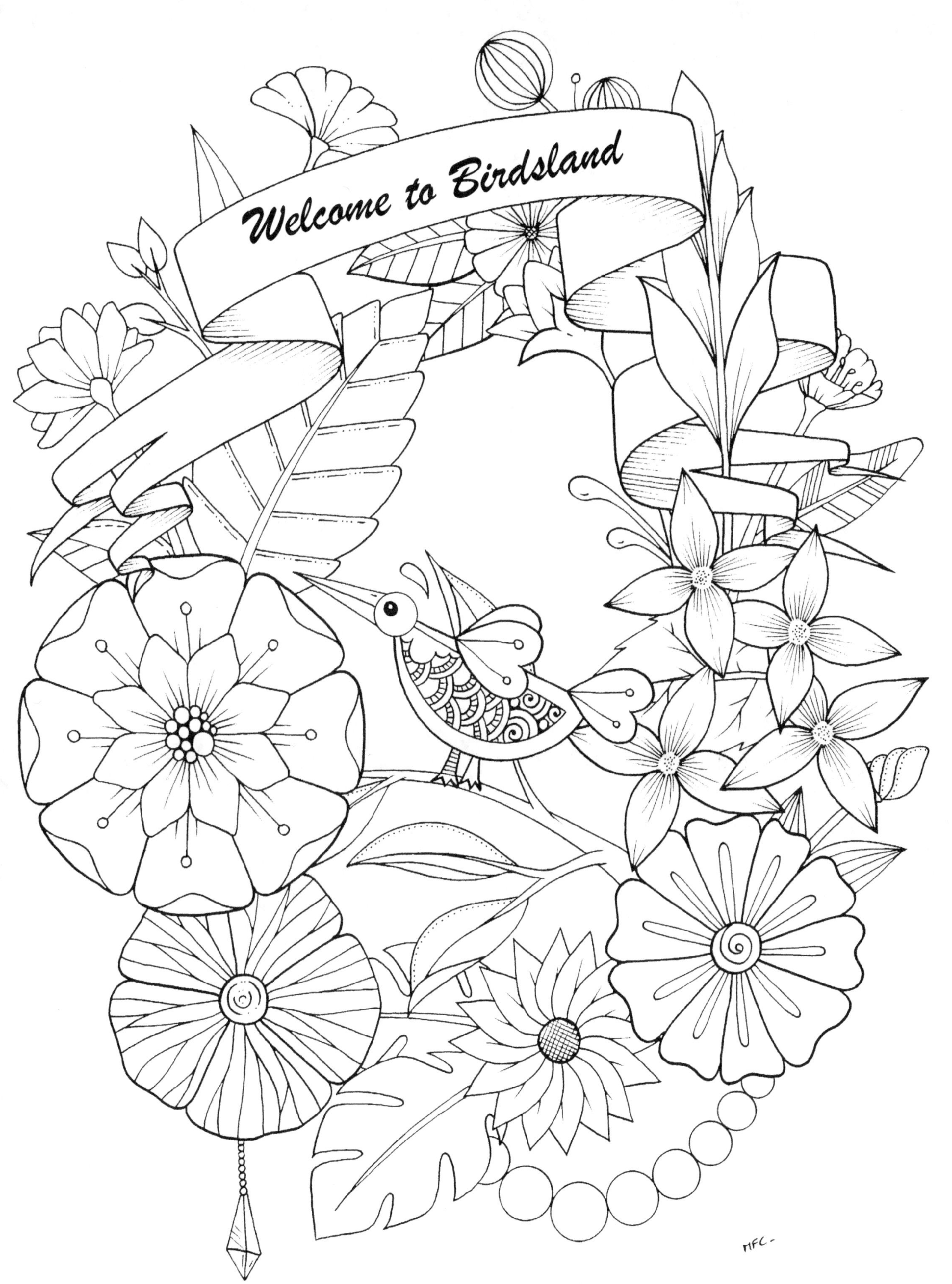

Welcome to Birdsland
MFC

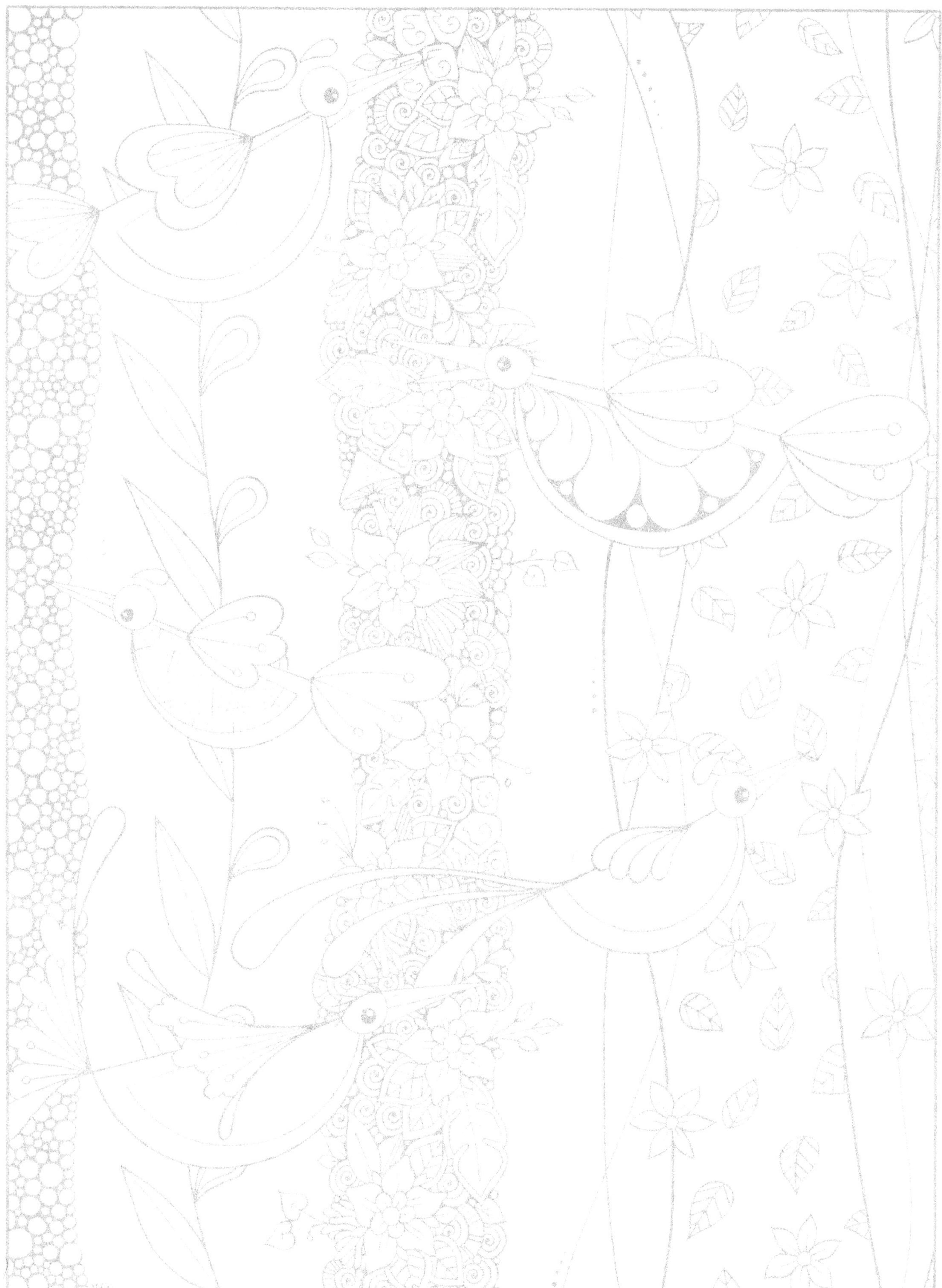

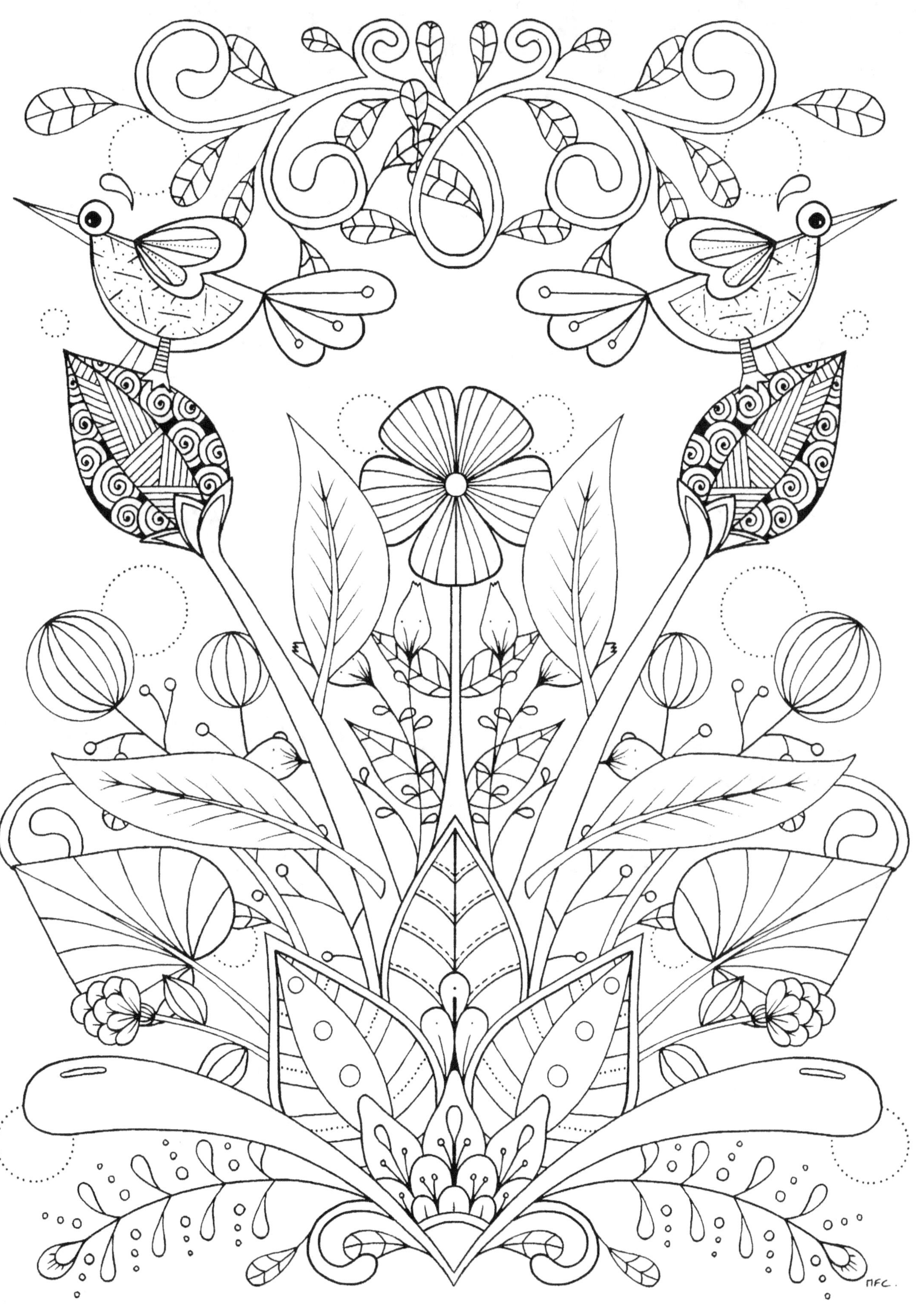

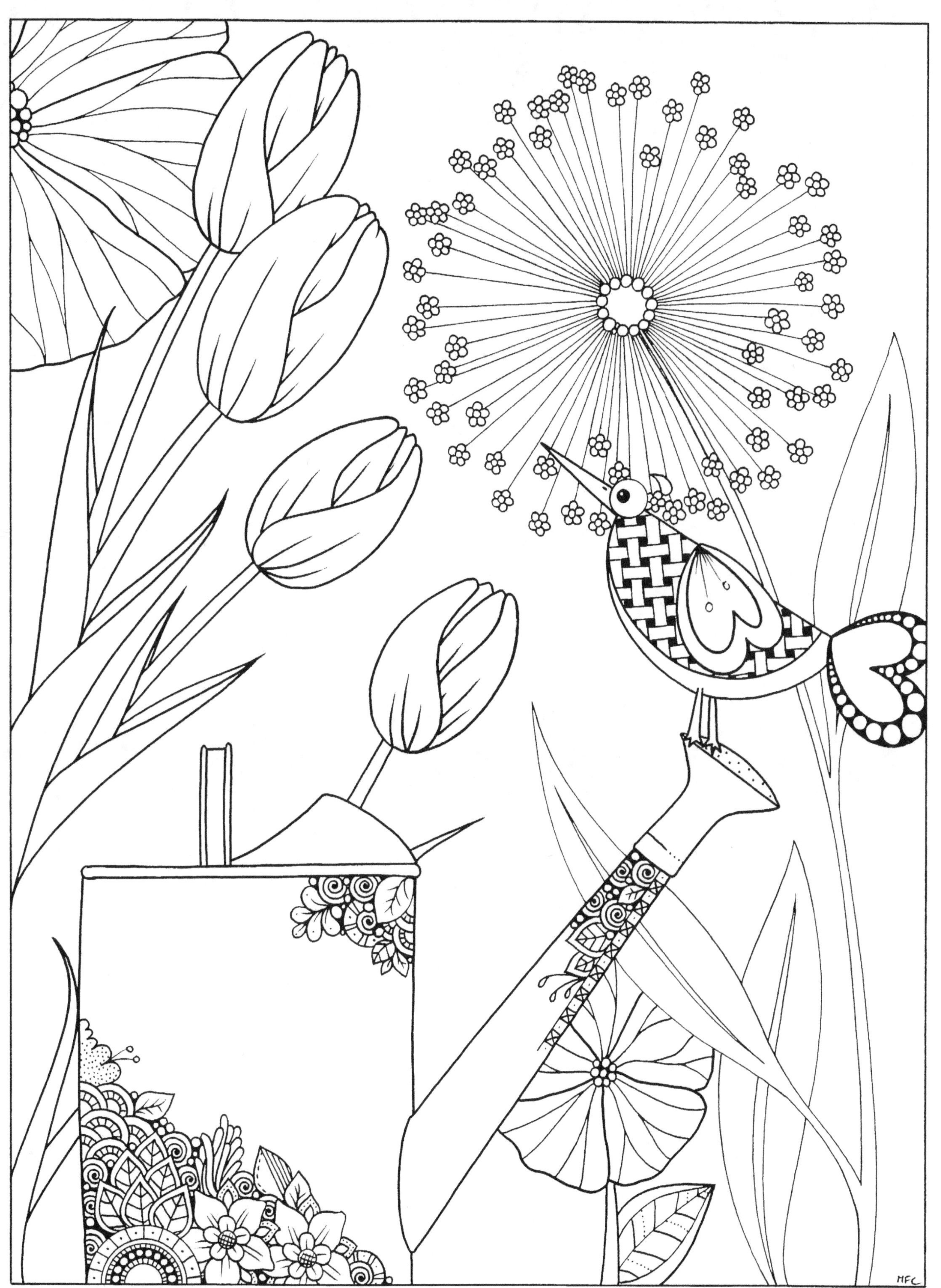

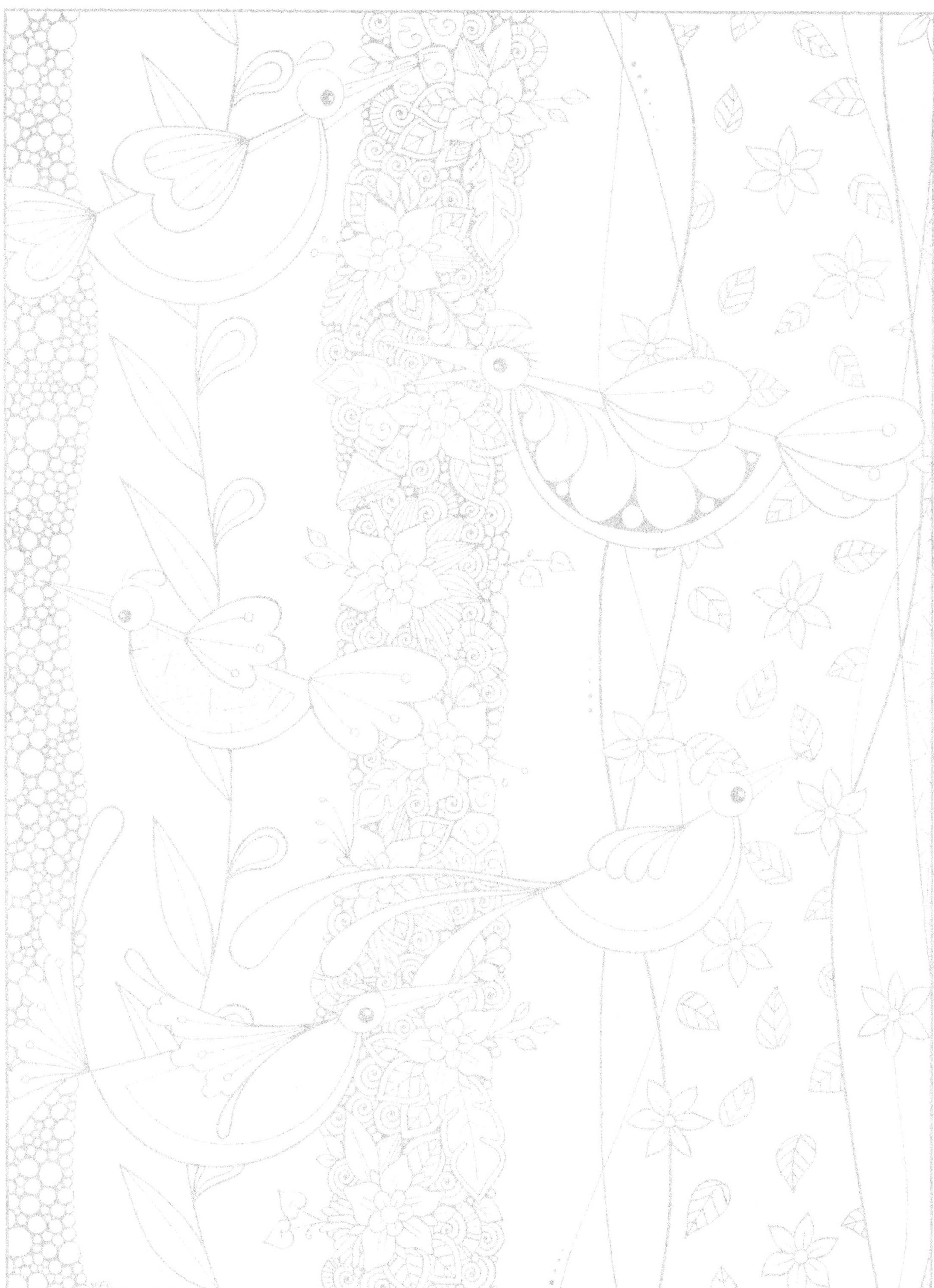

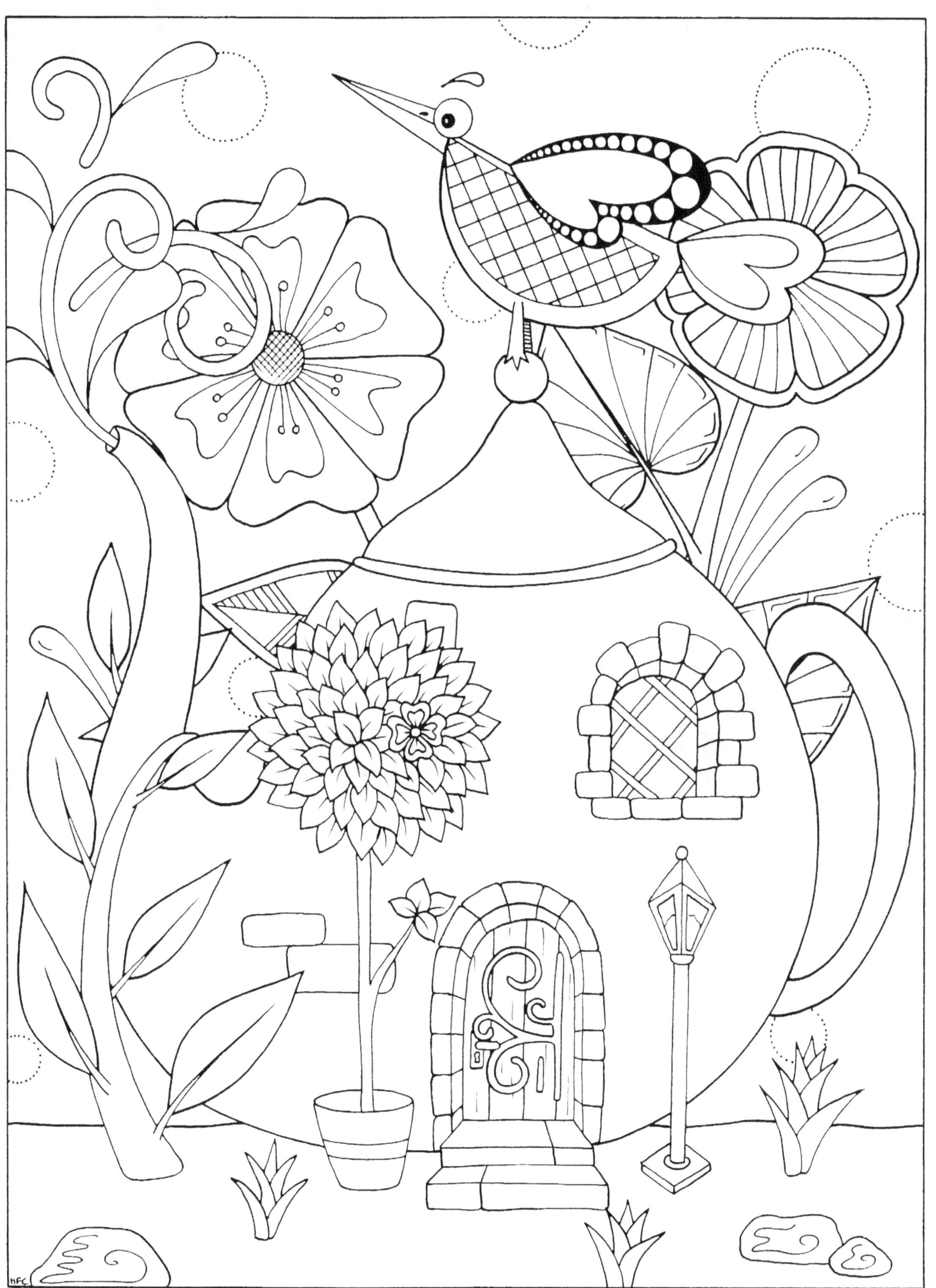

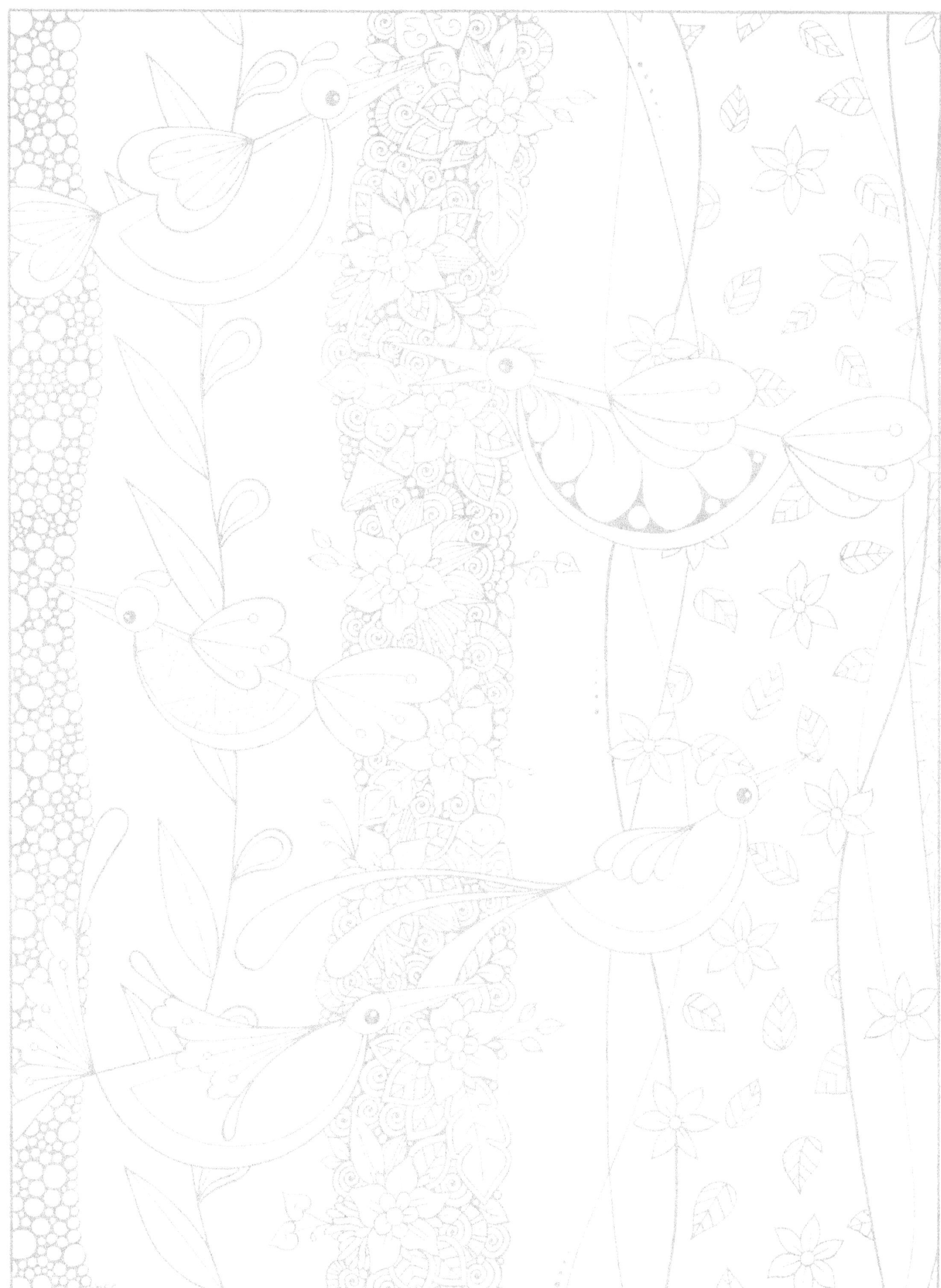

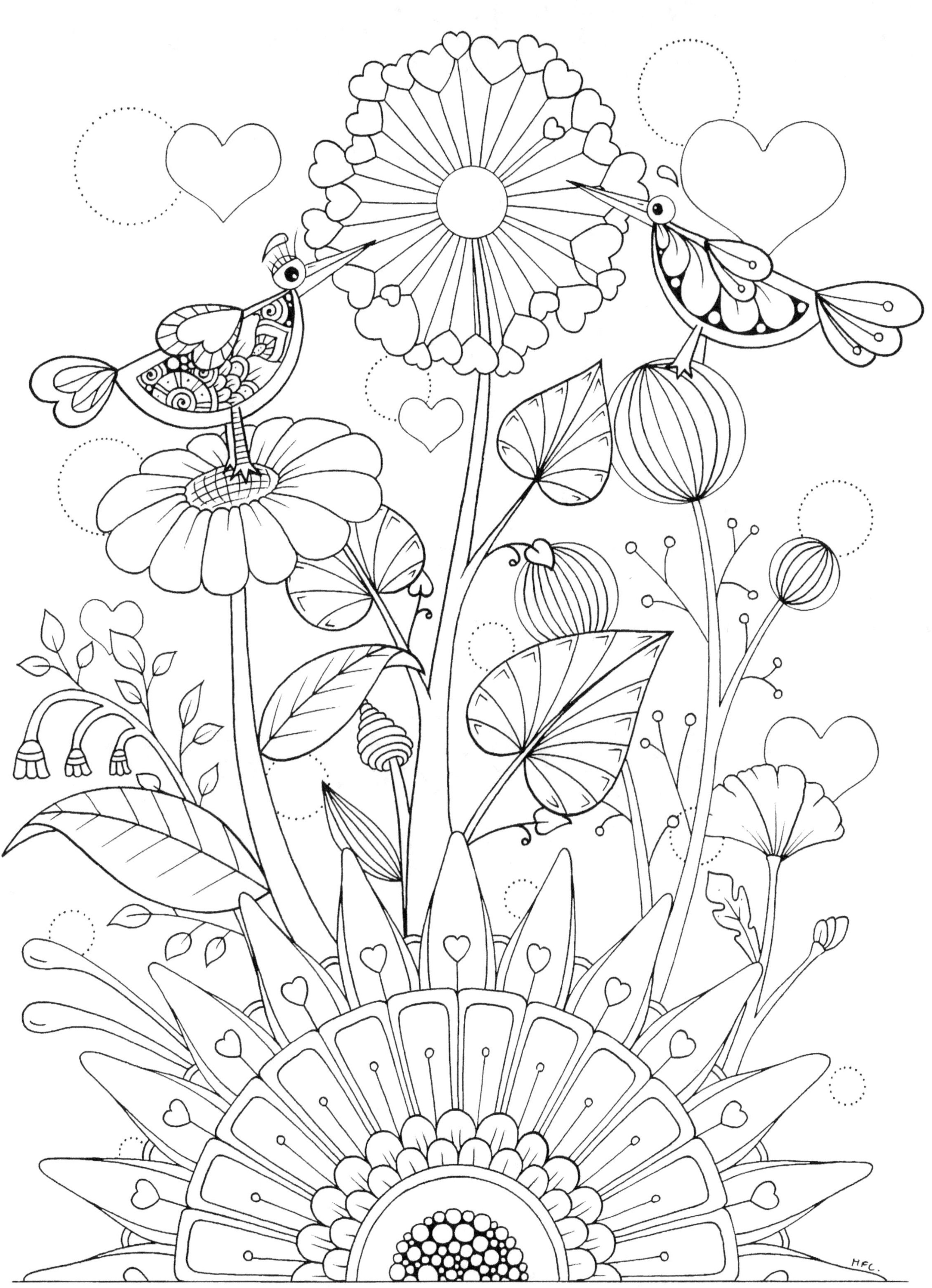

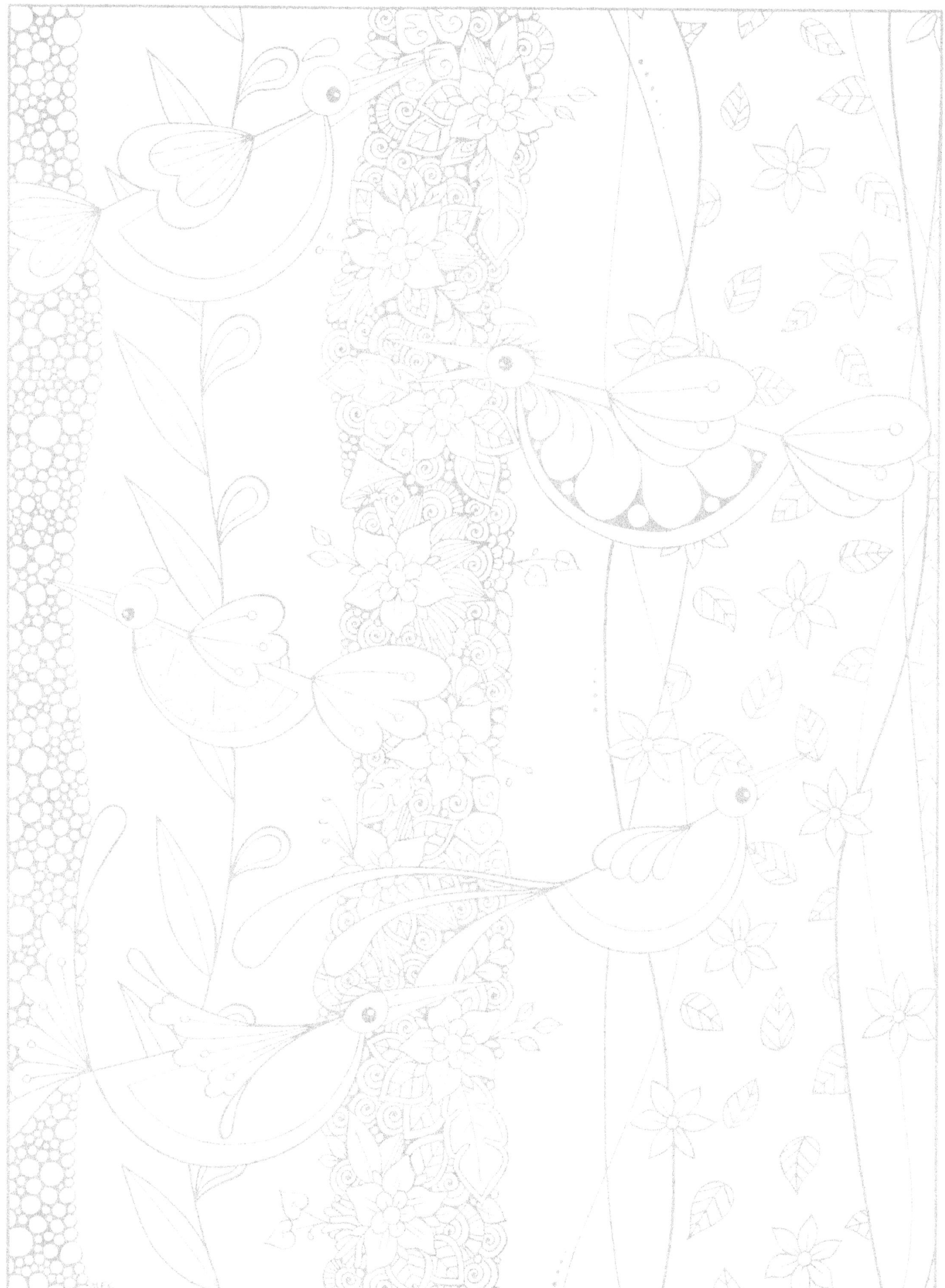

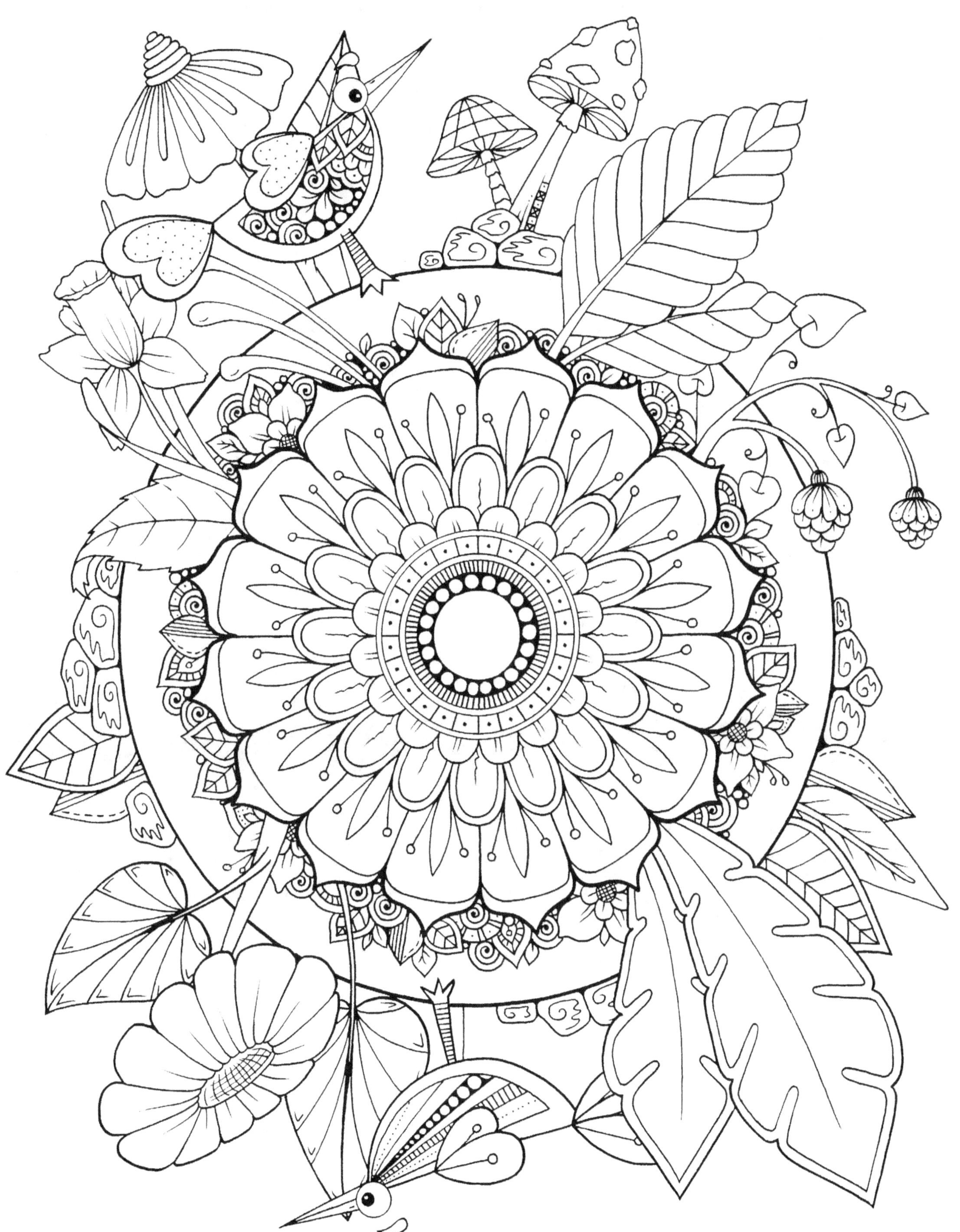

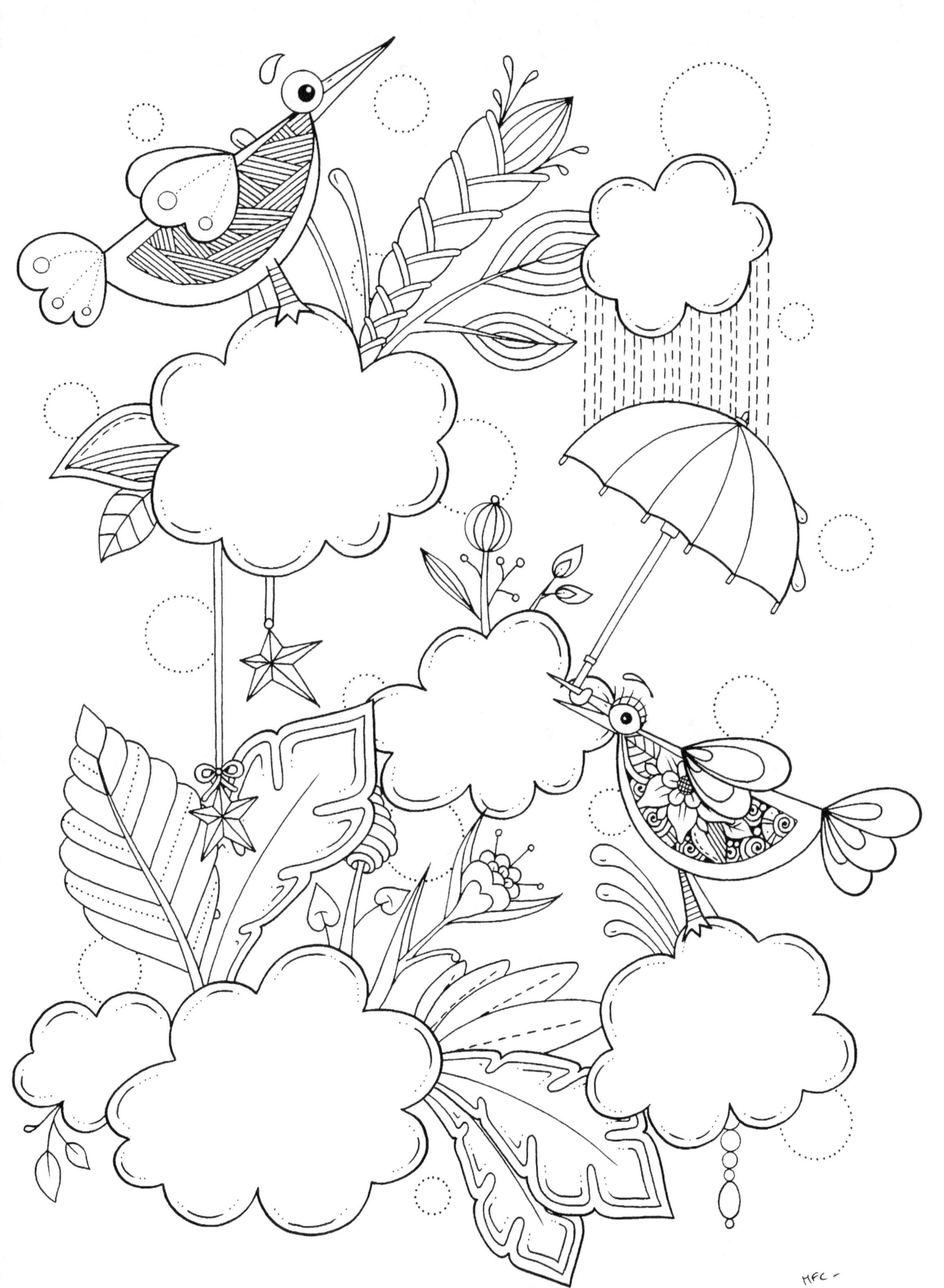

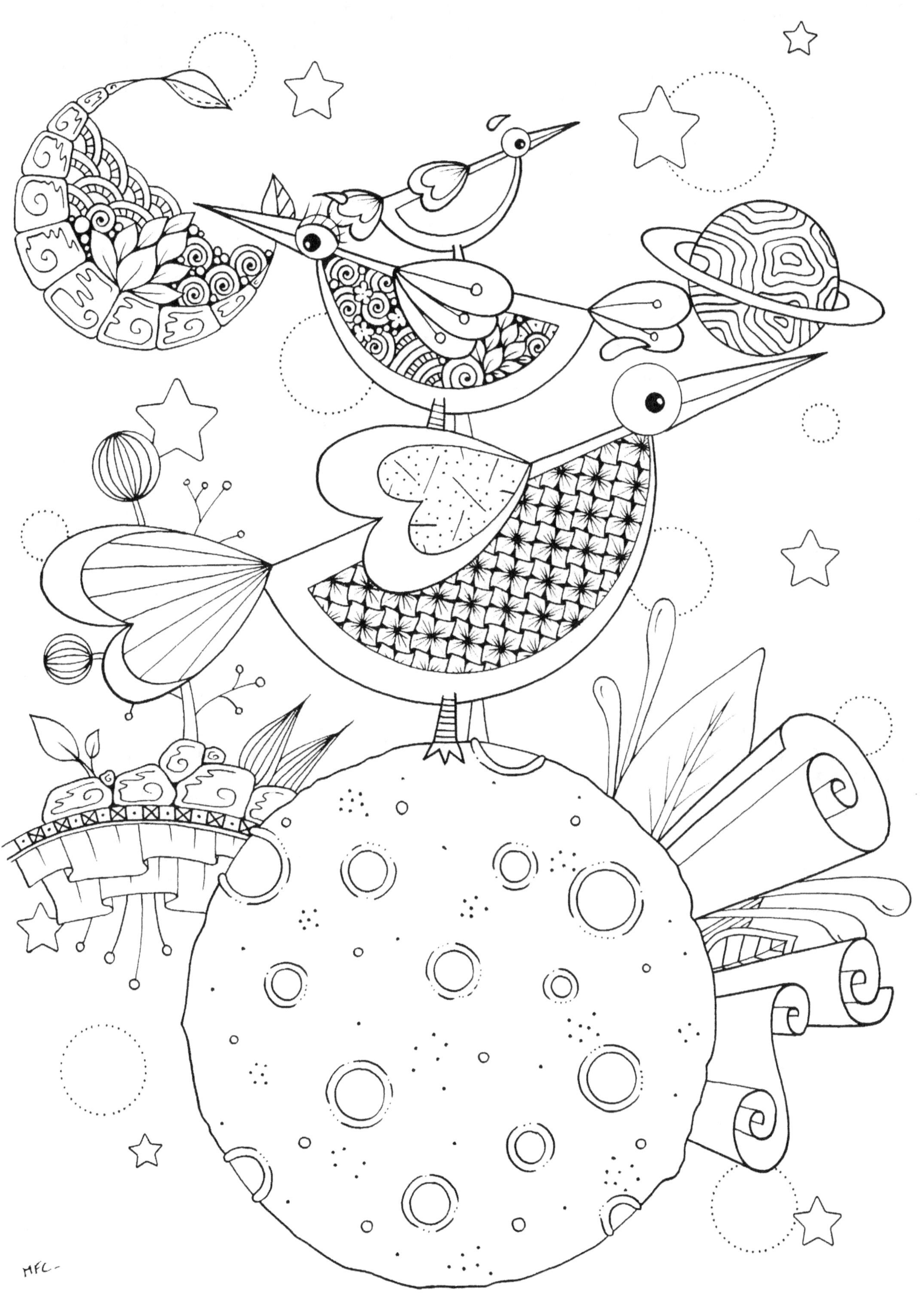

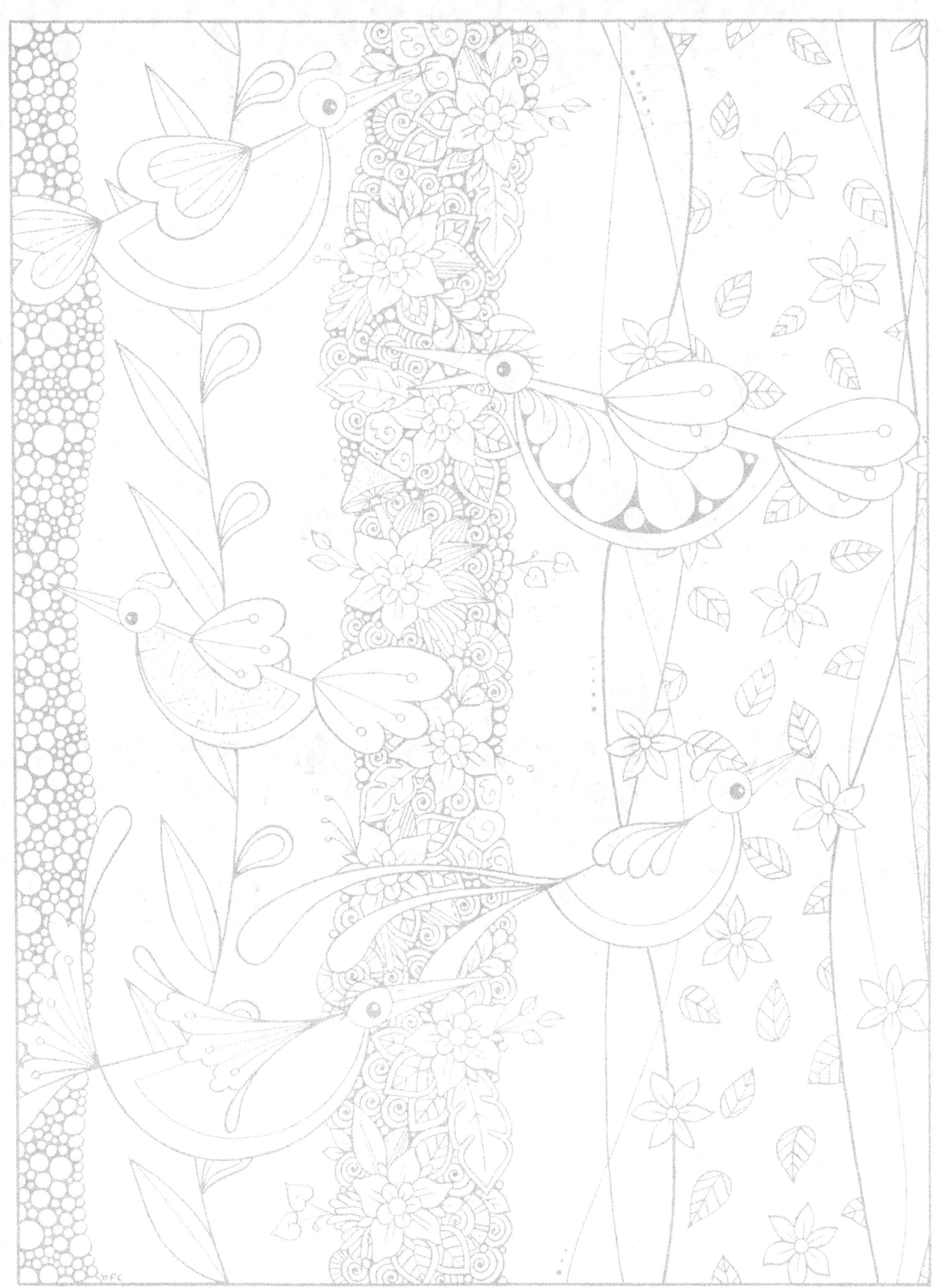

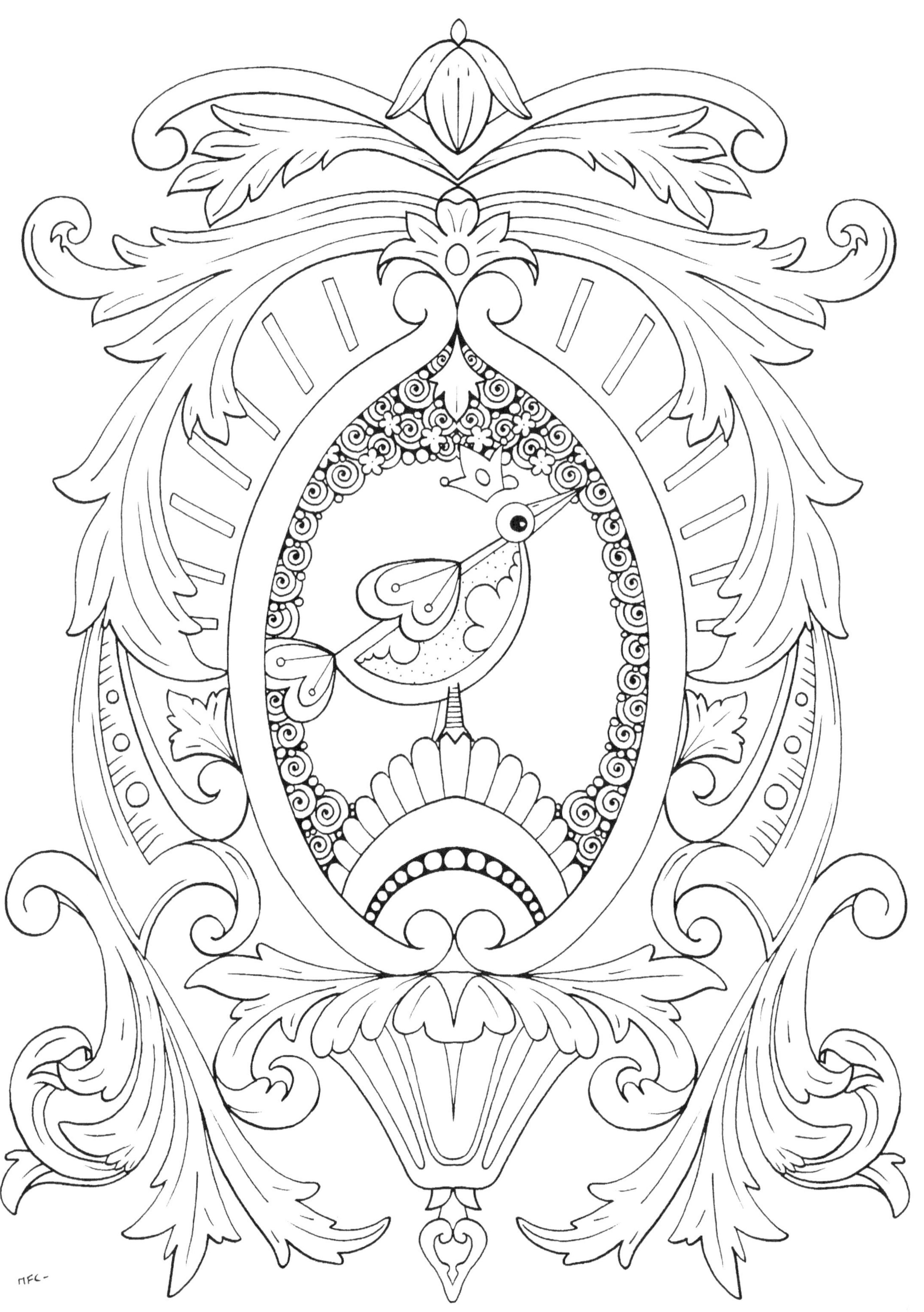

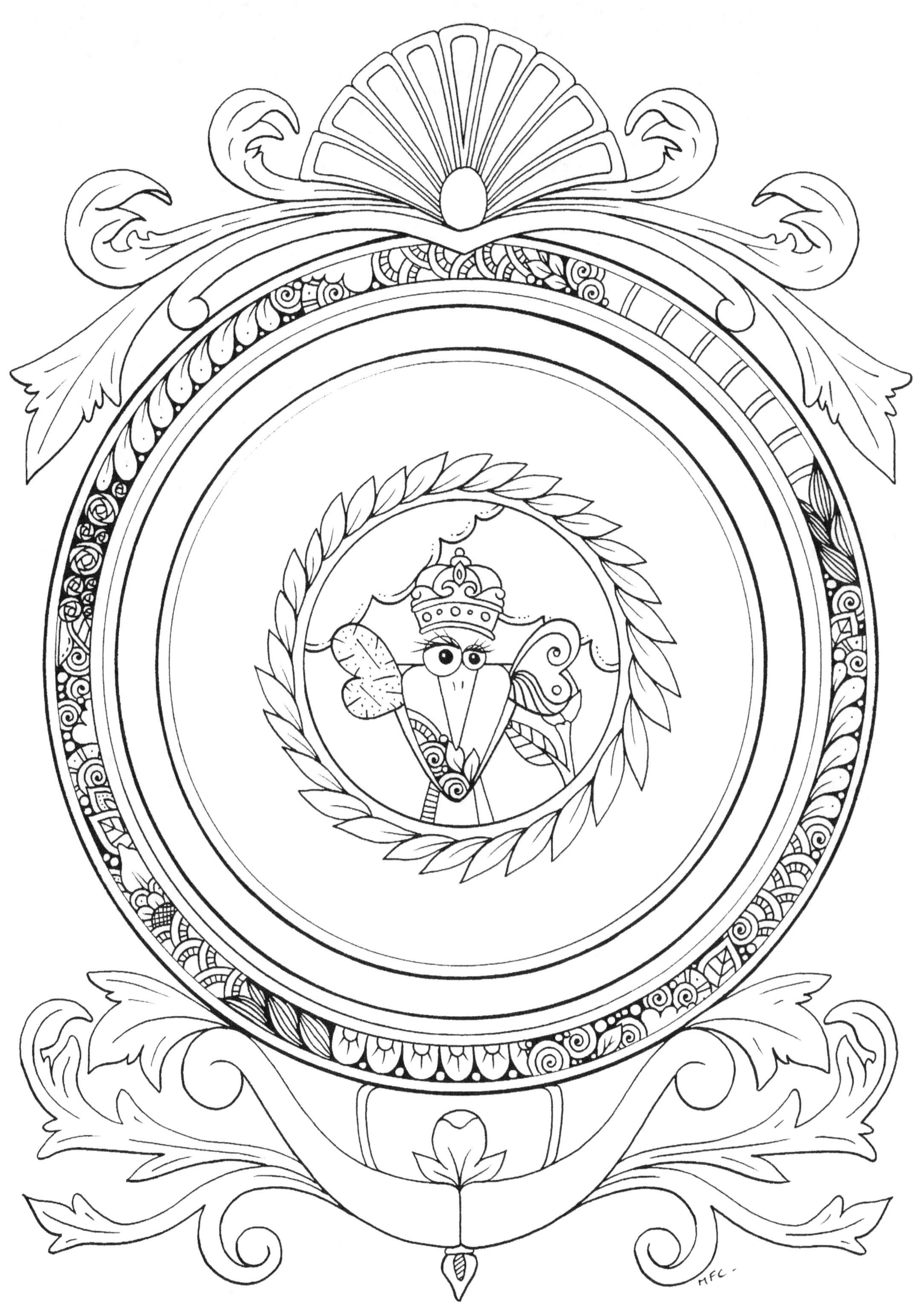

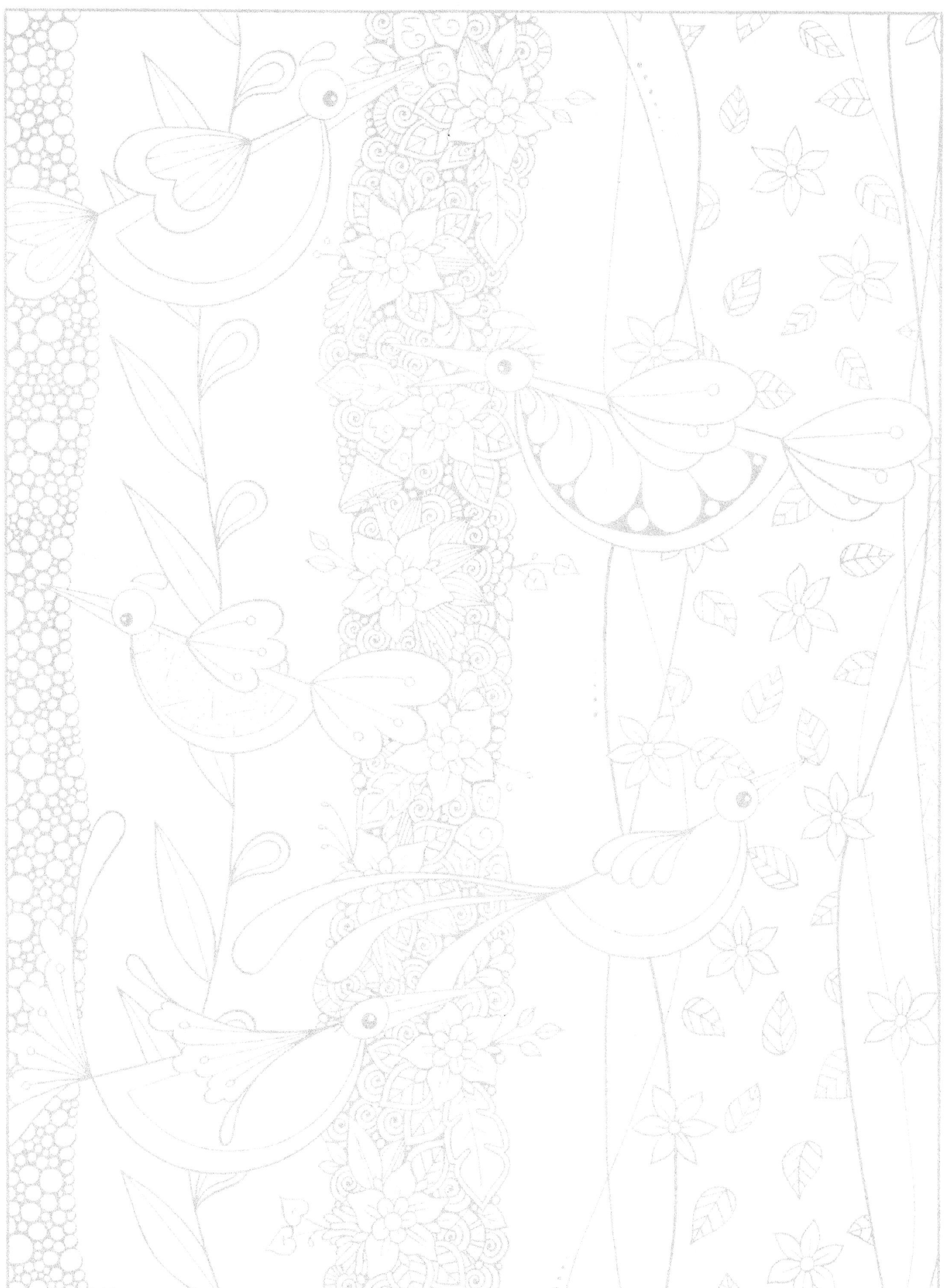

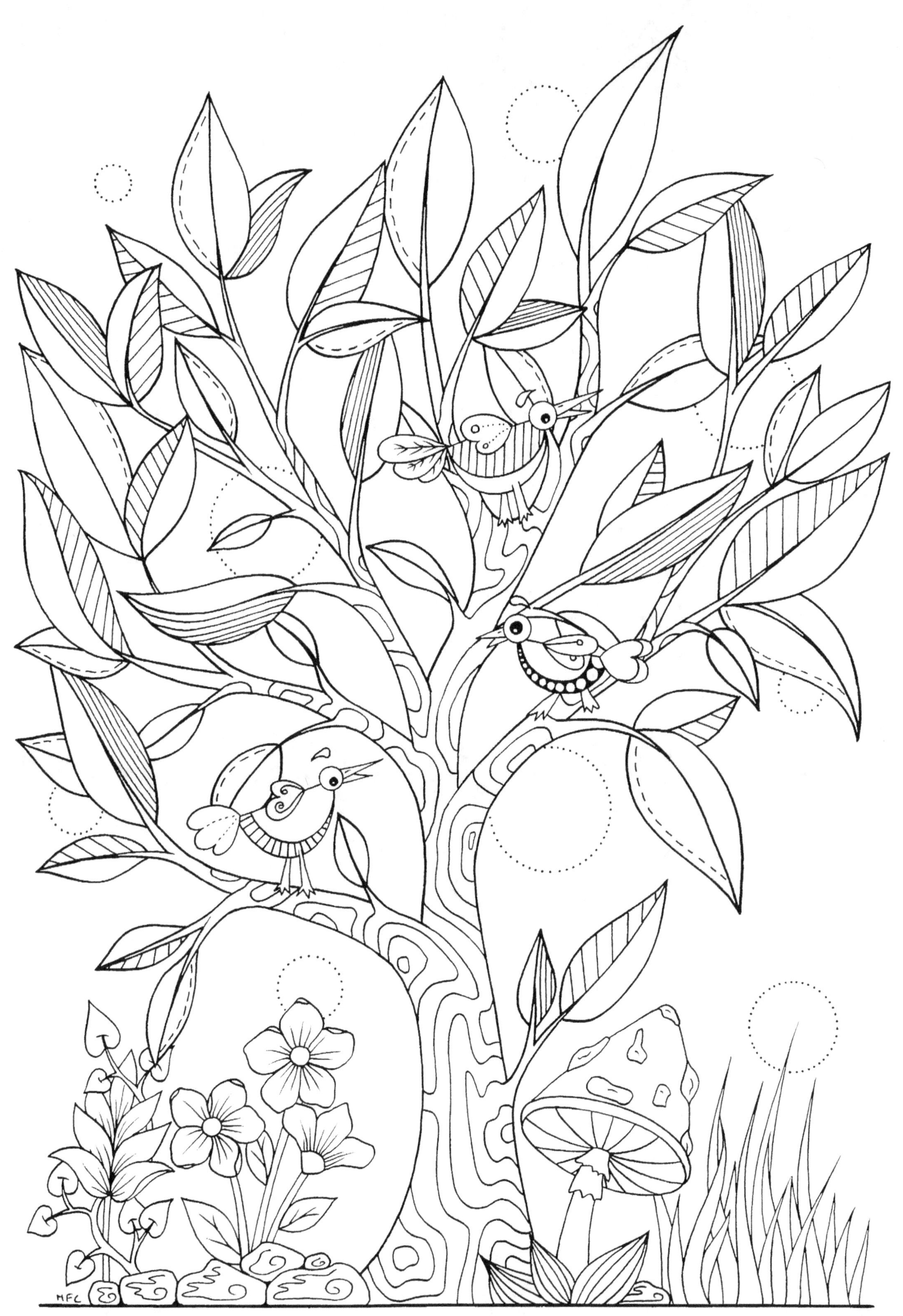

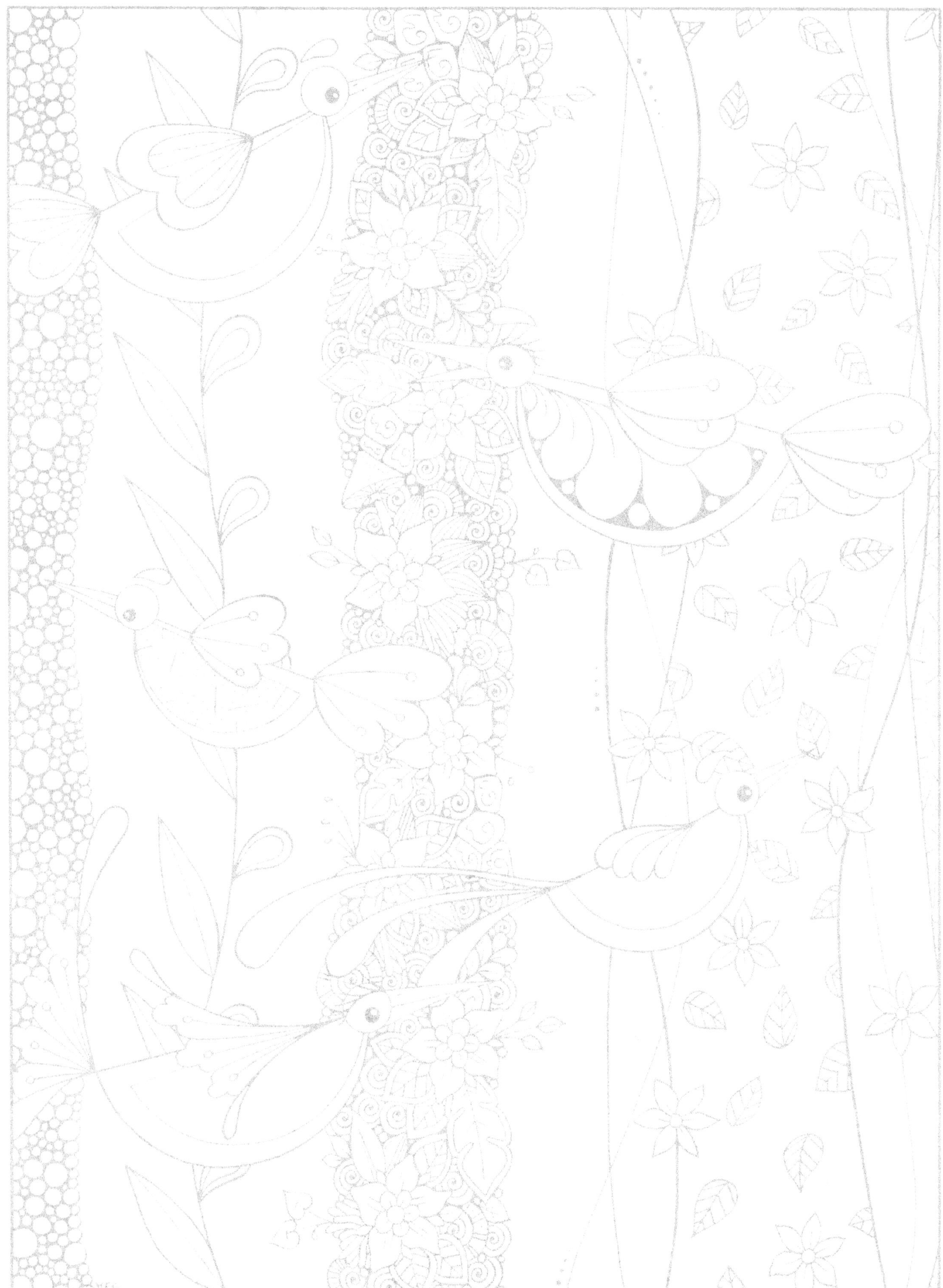

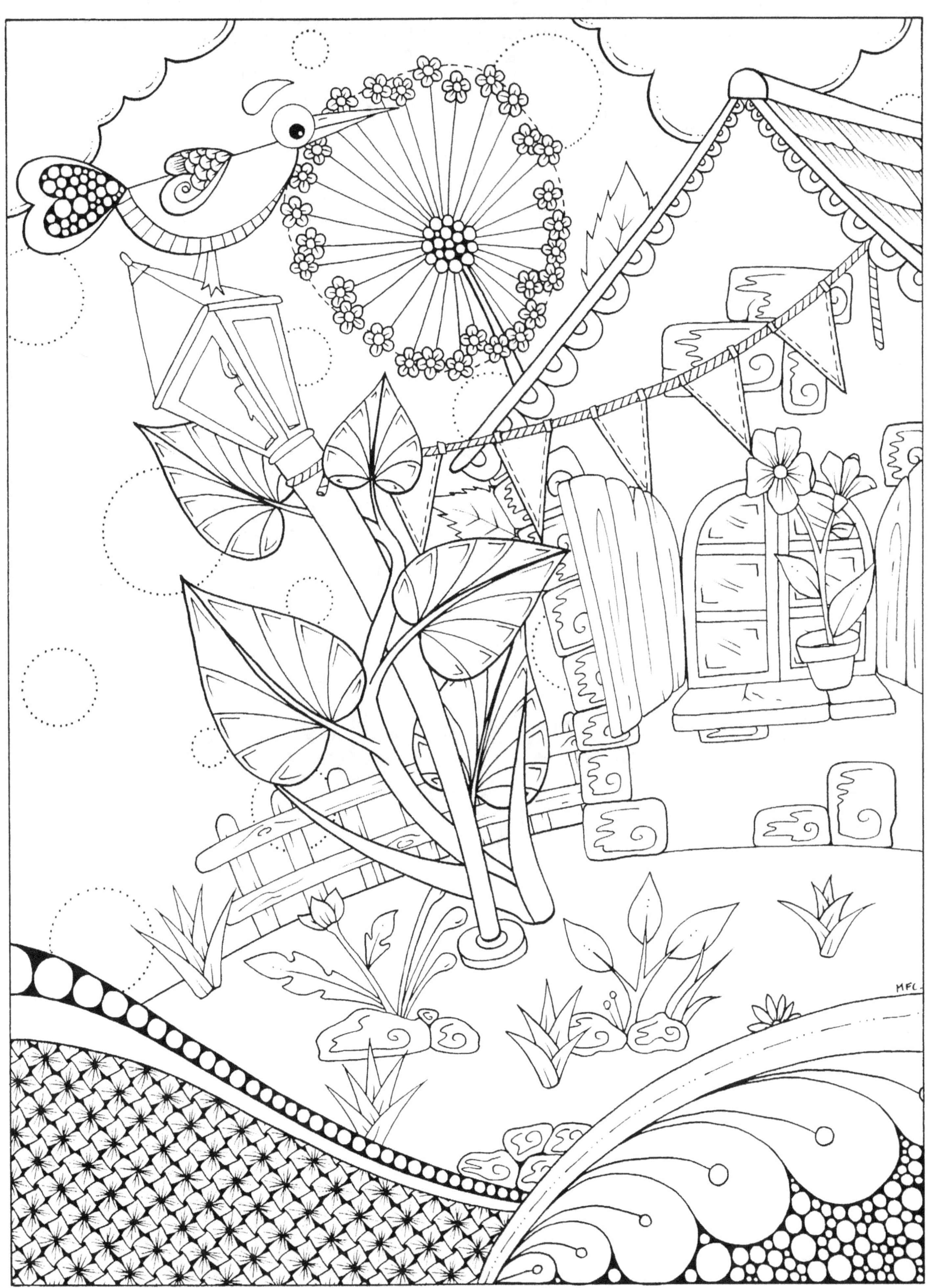

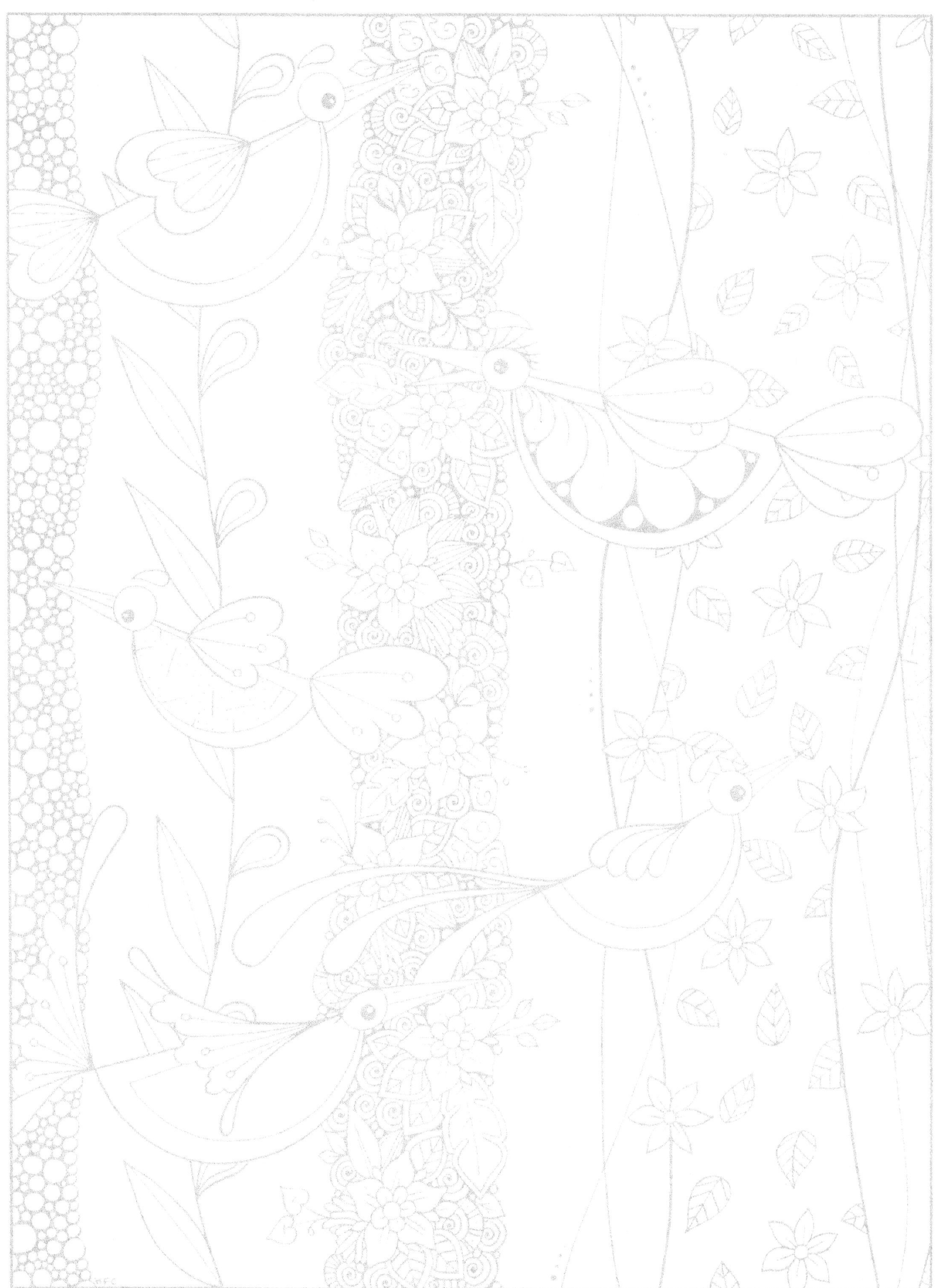

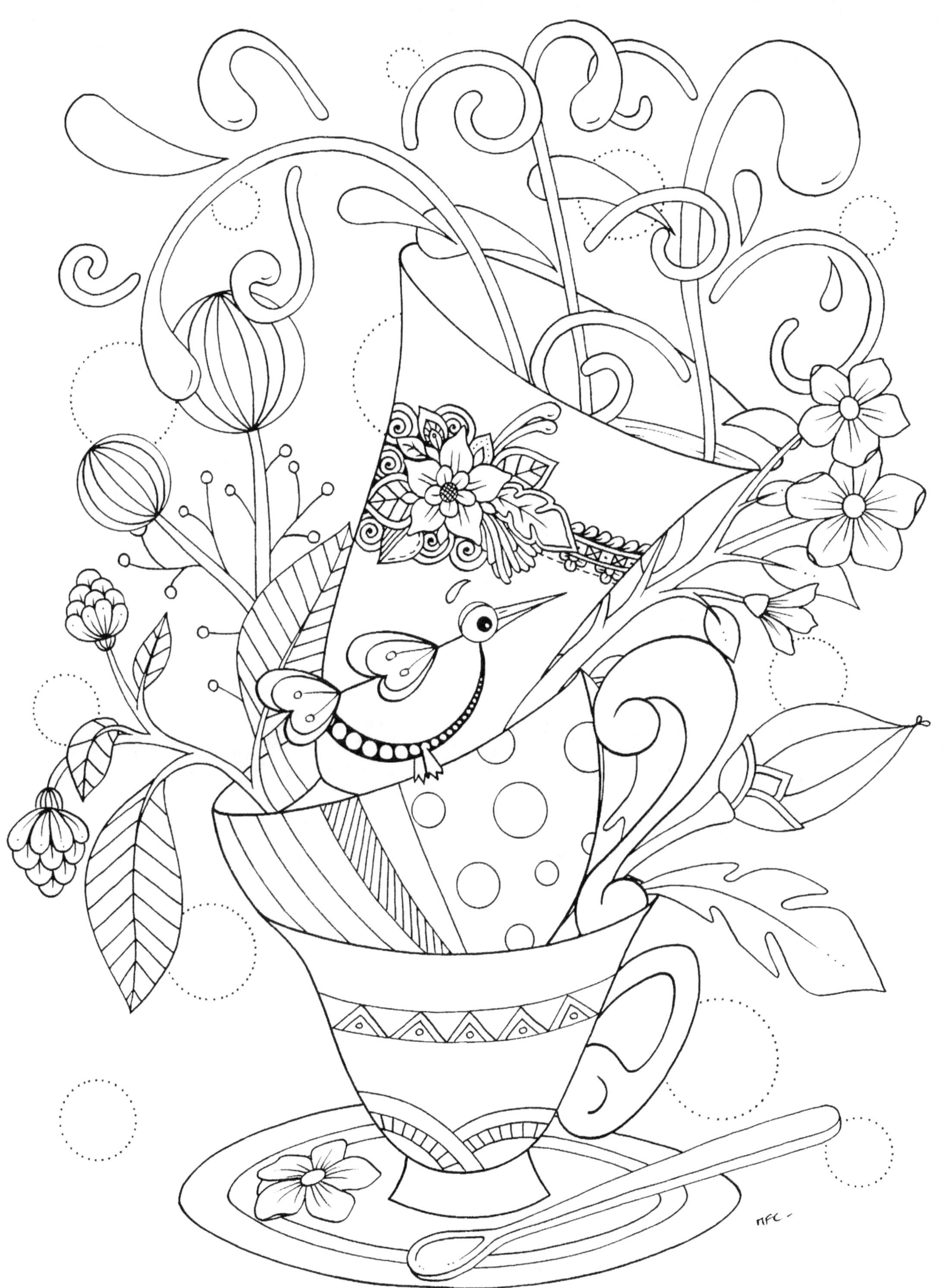

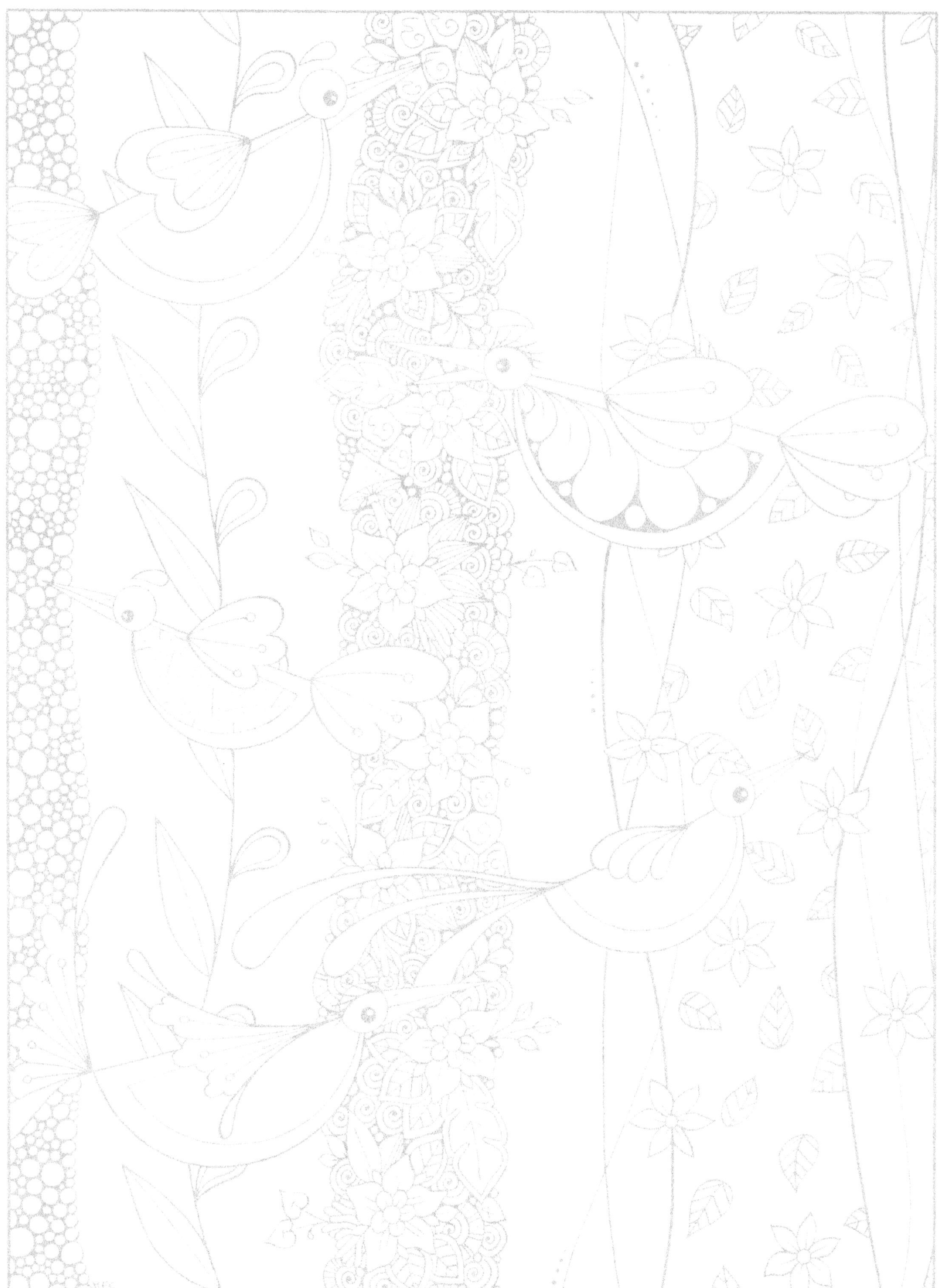

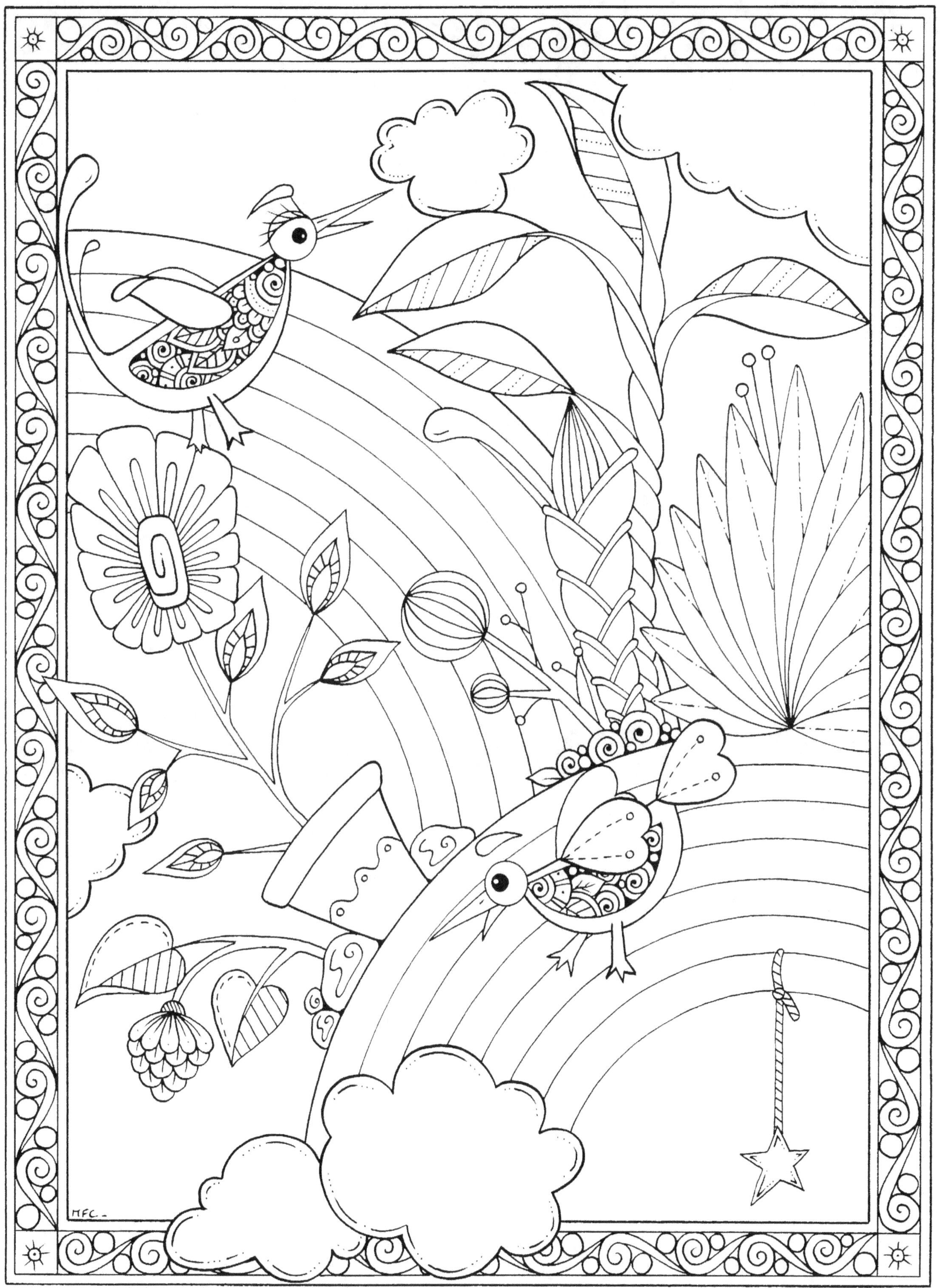

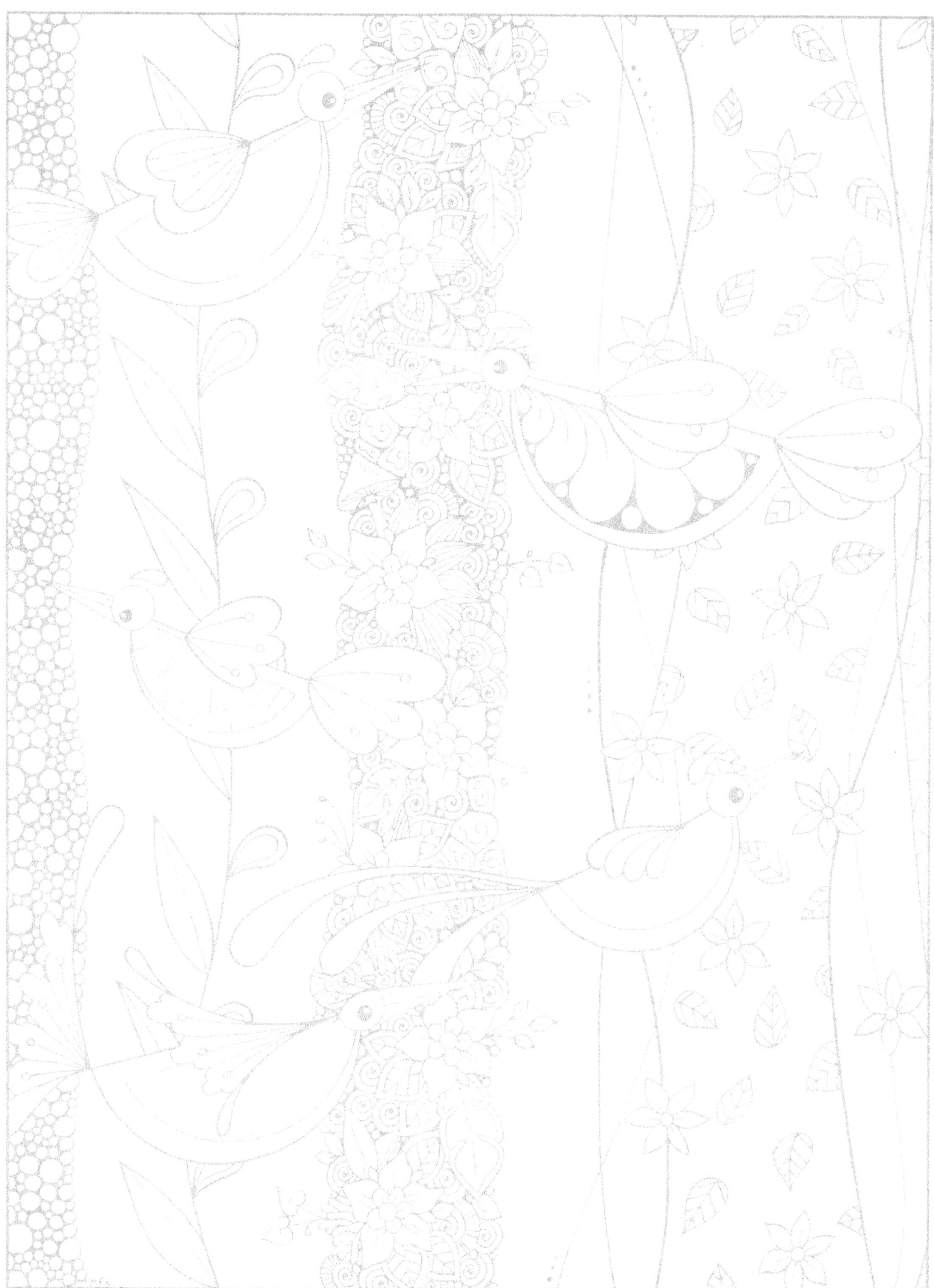

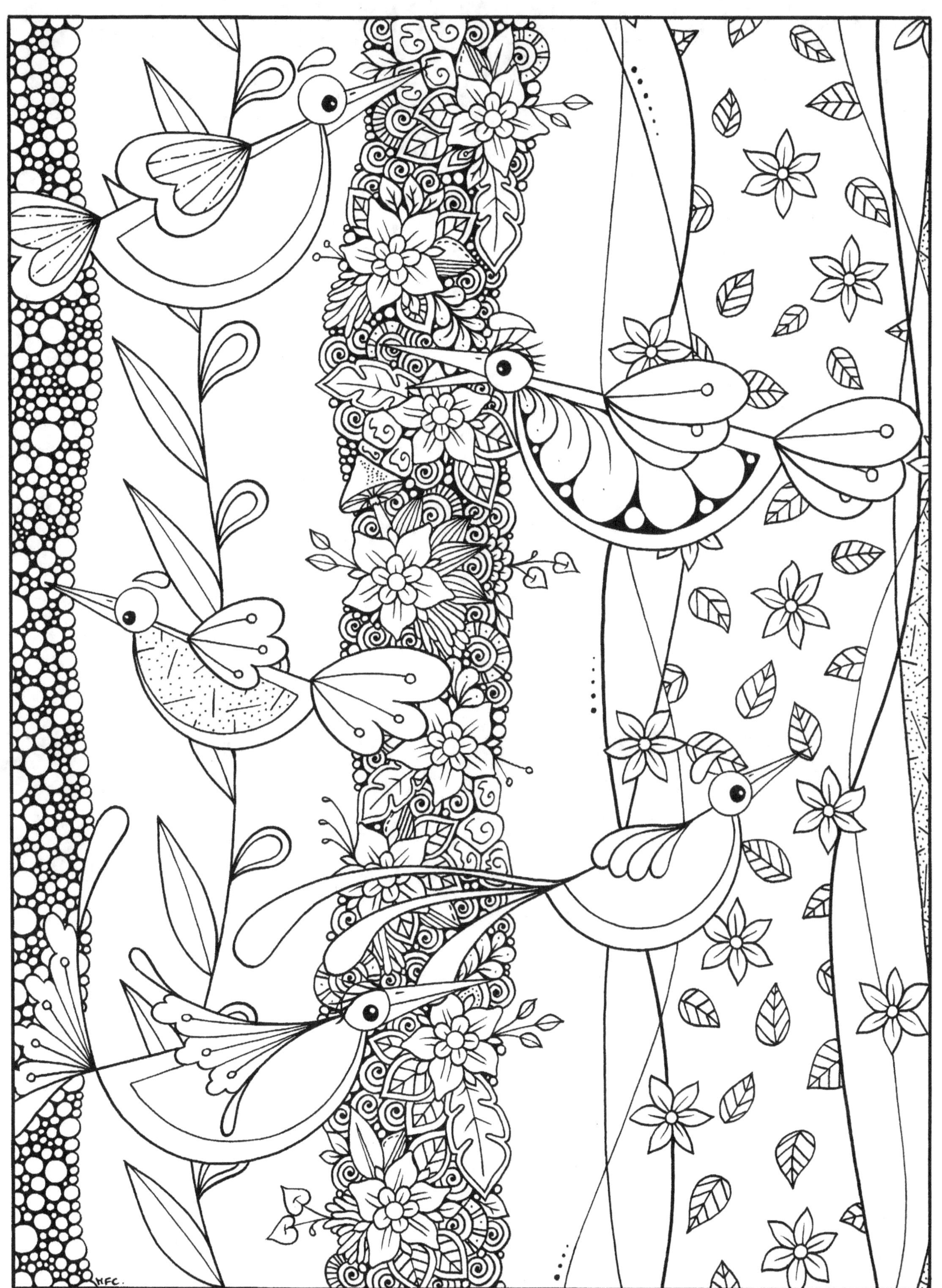

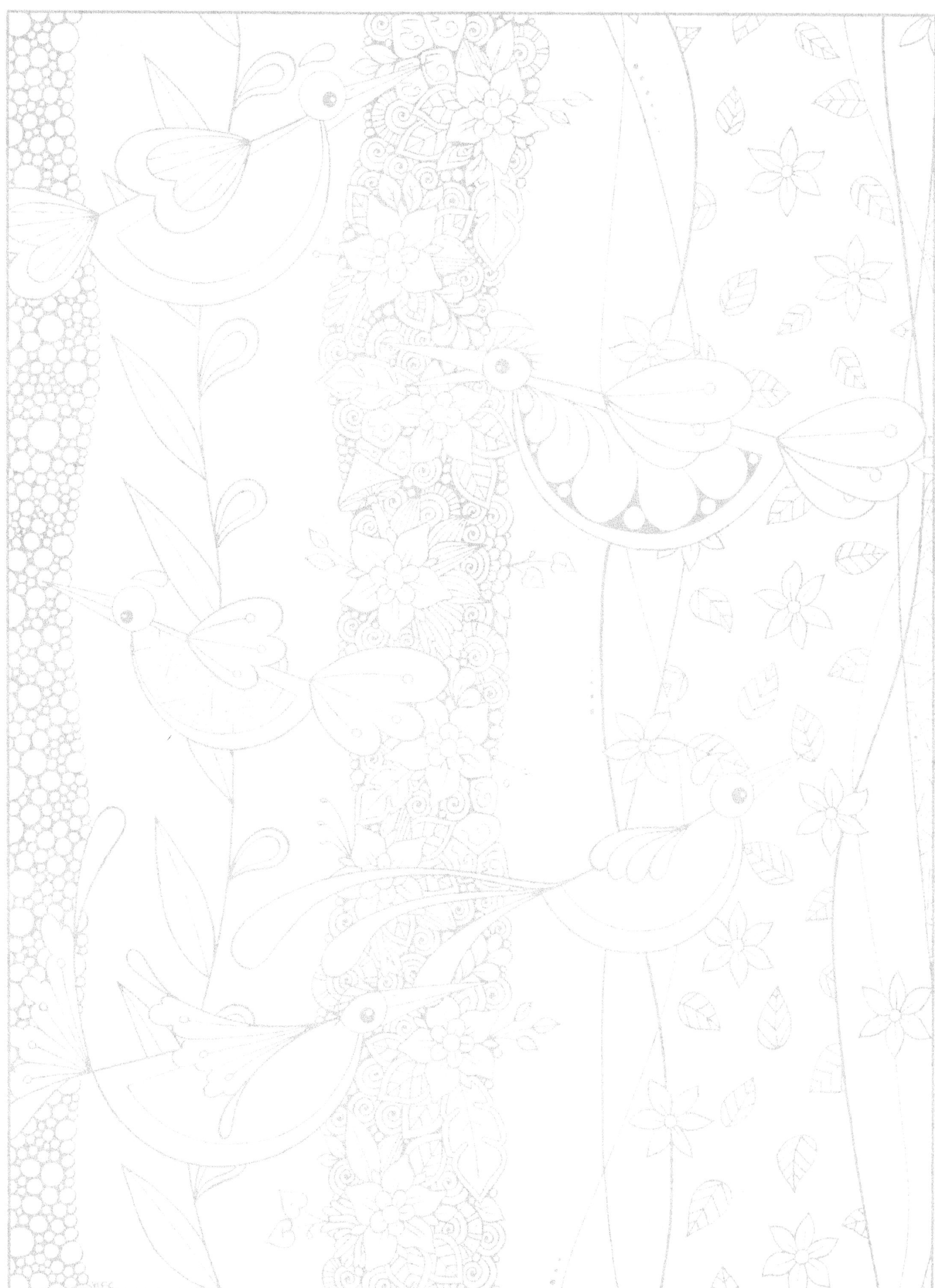

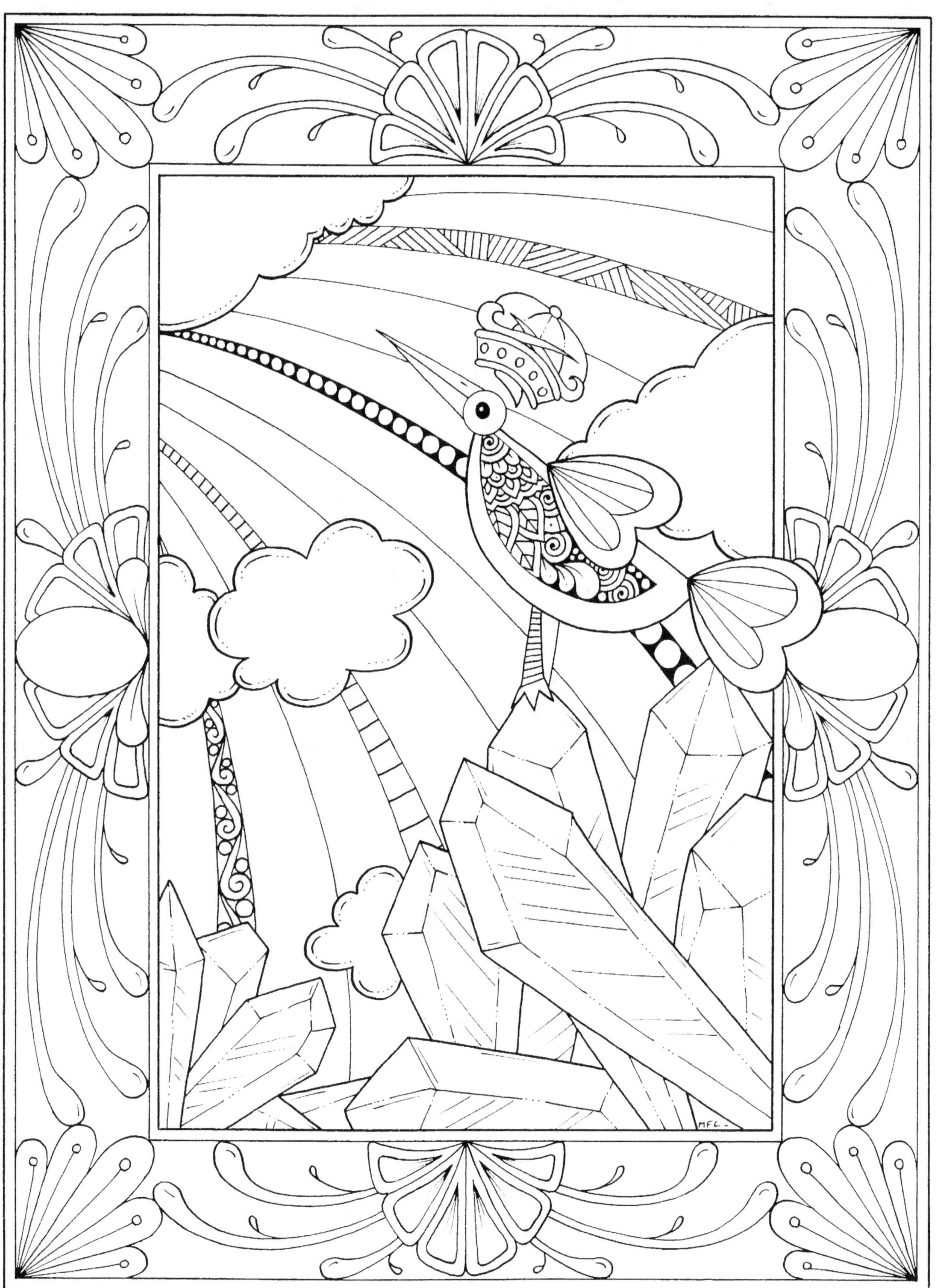

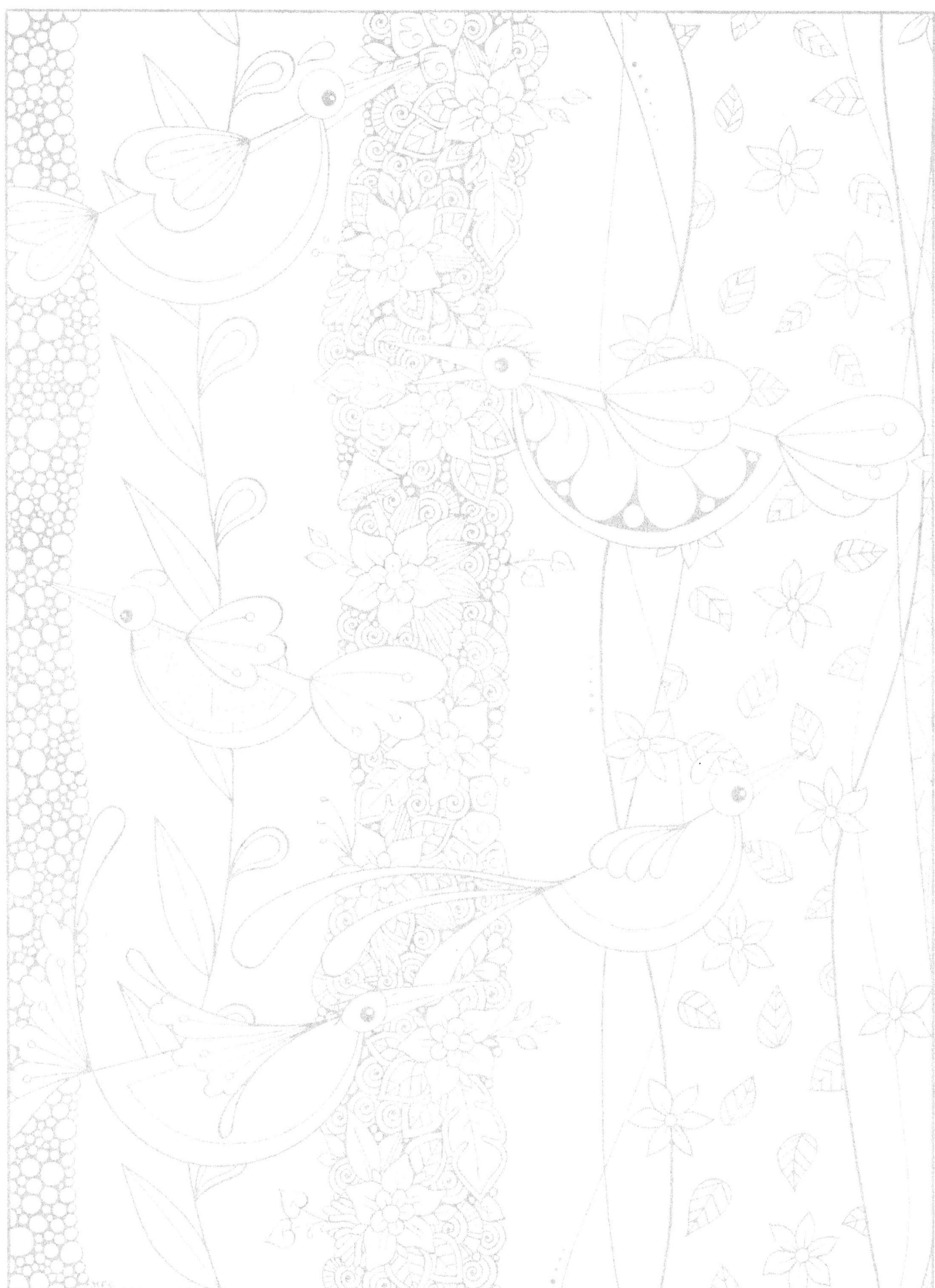

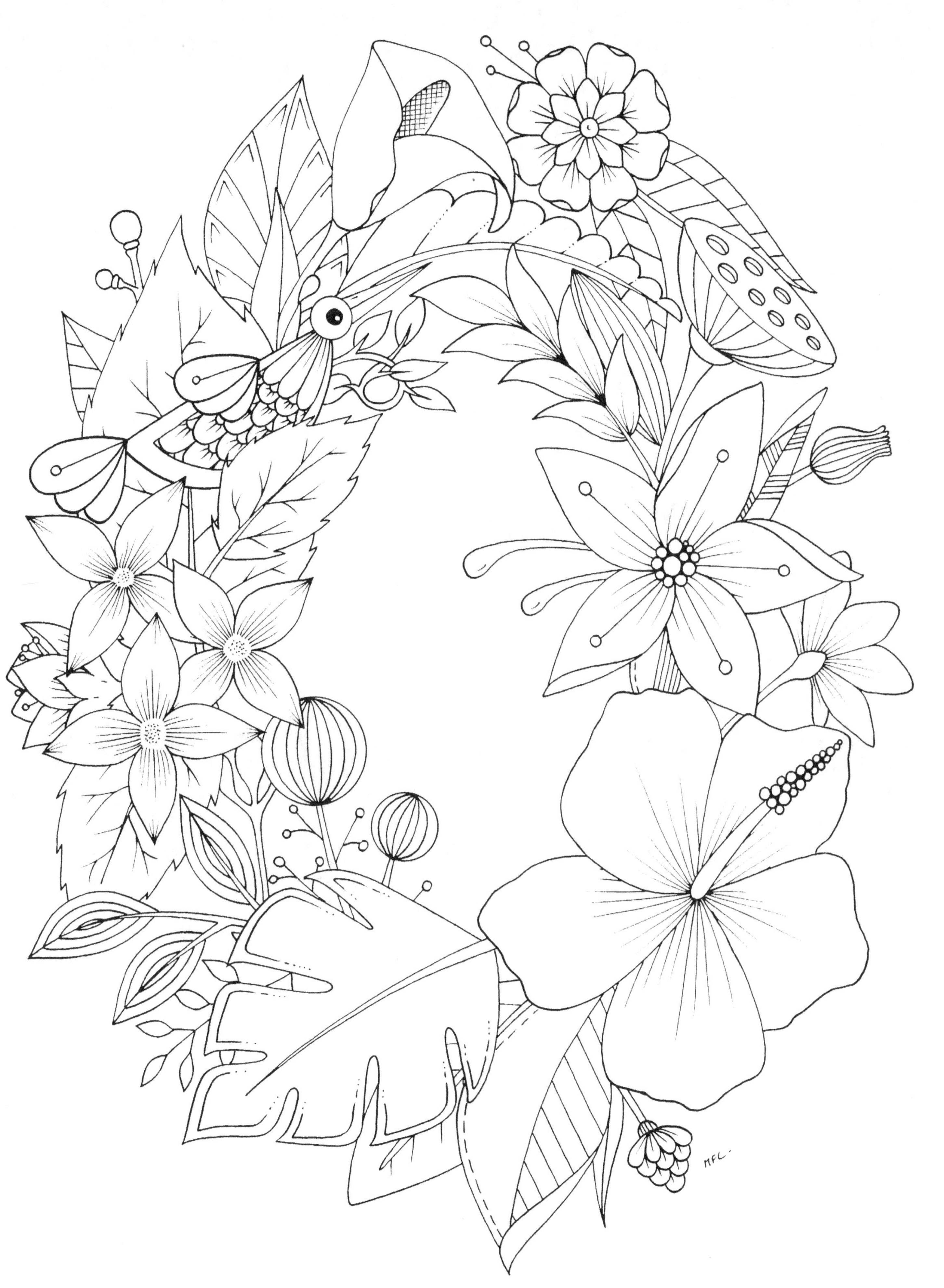

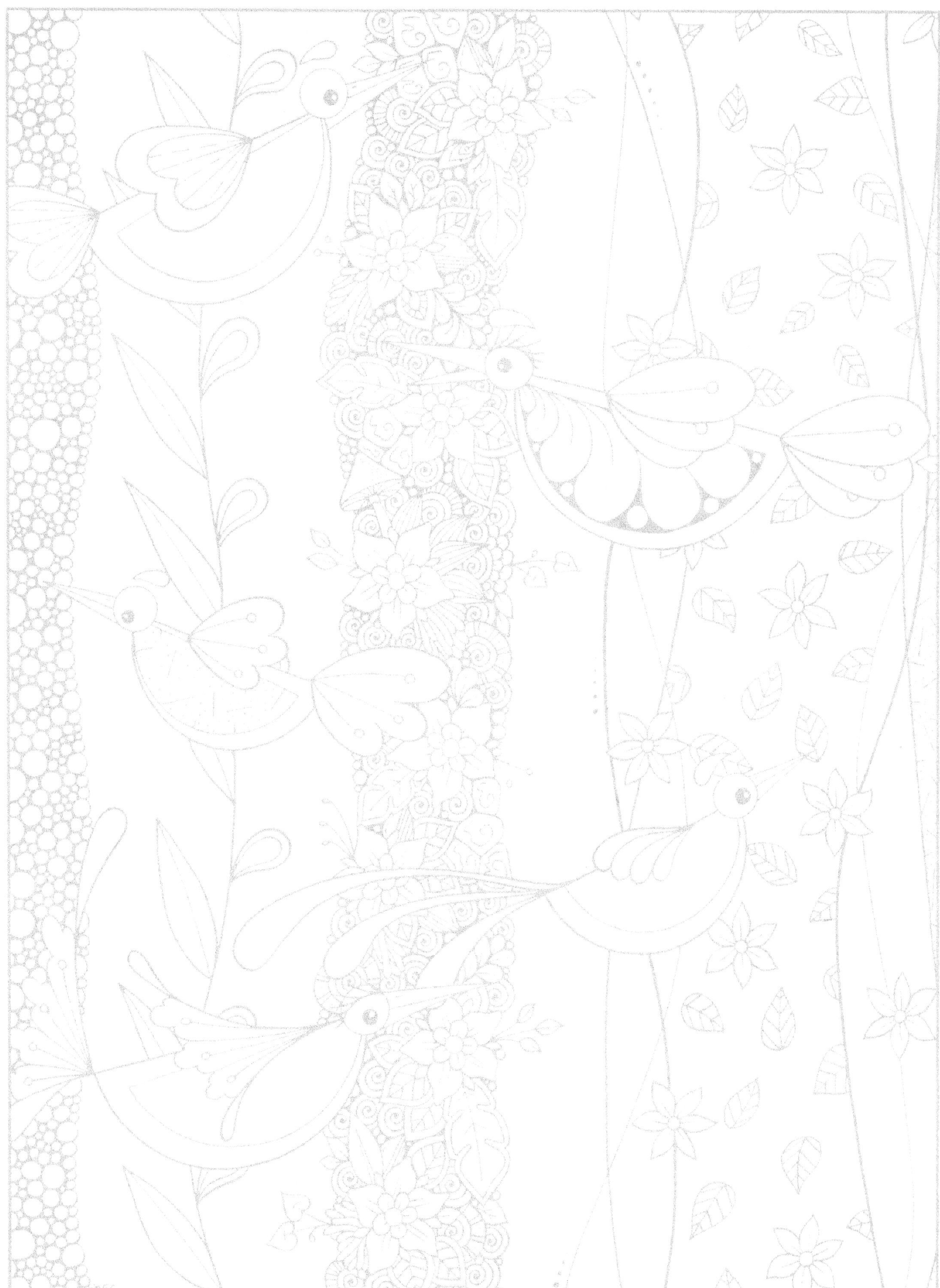

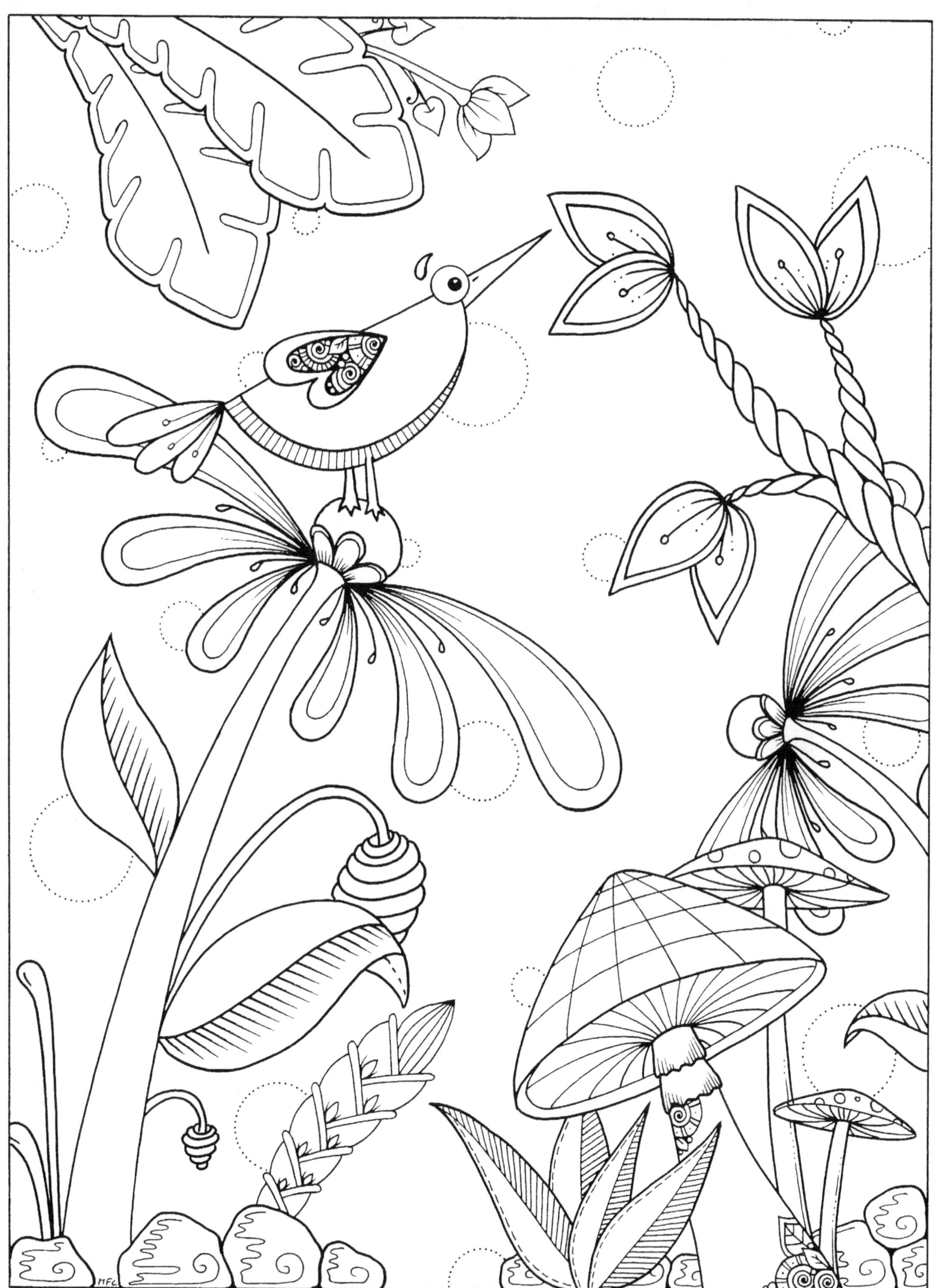

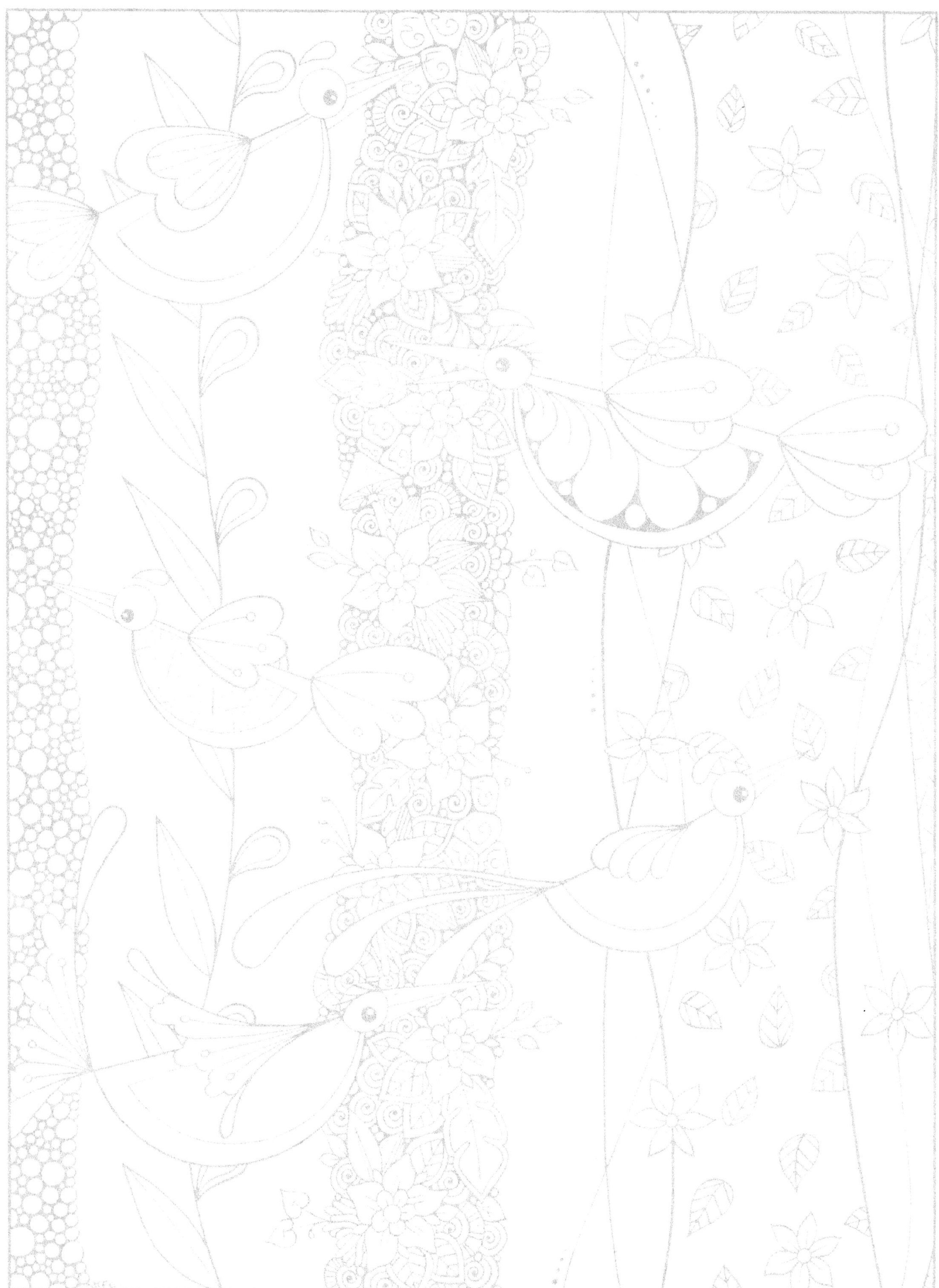

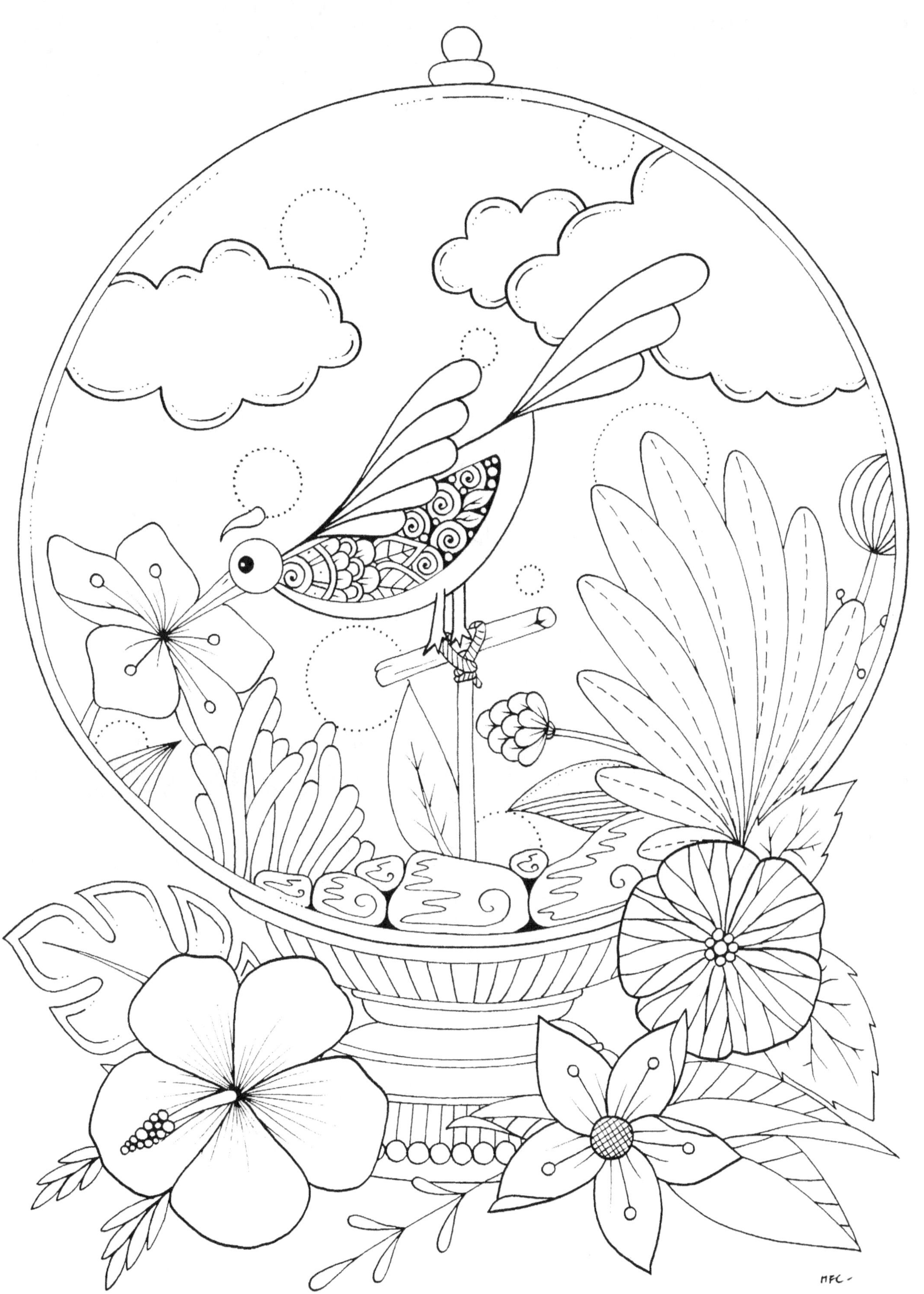
MFC

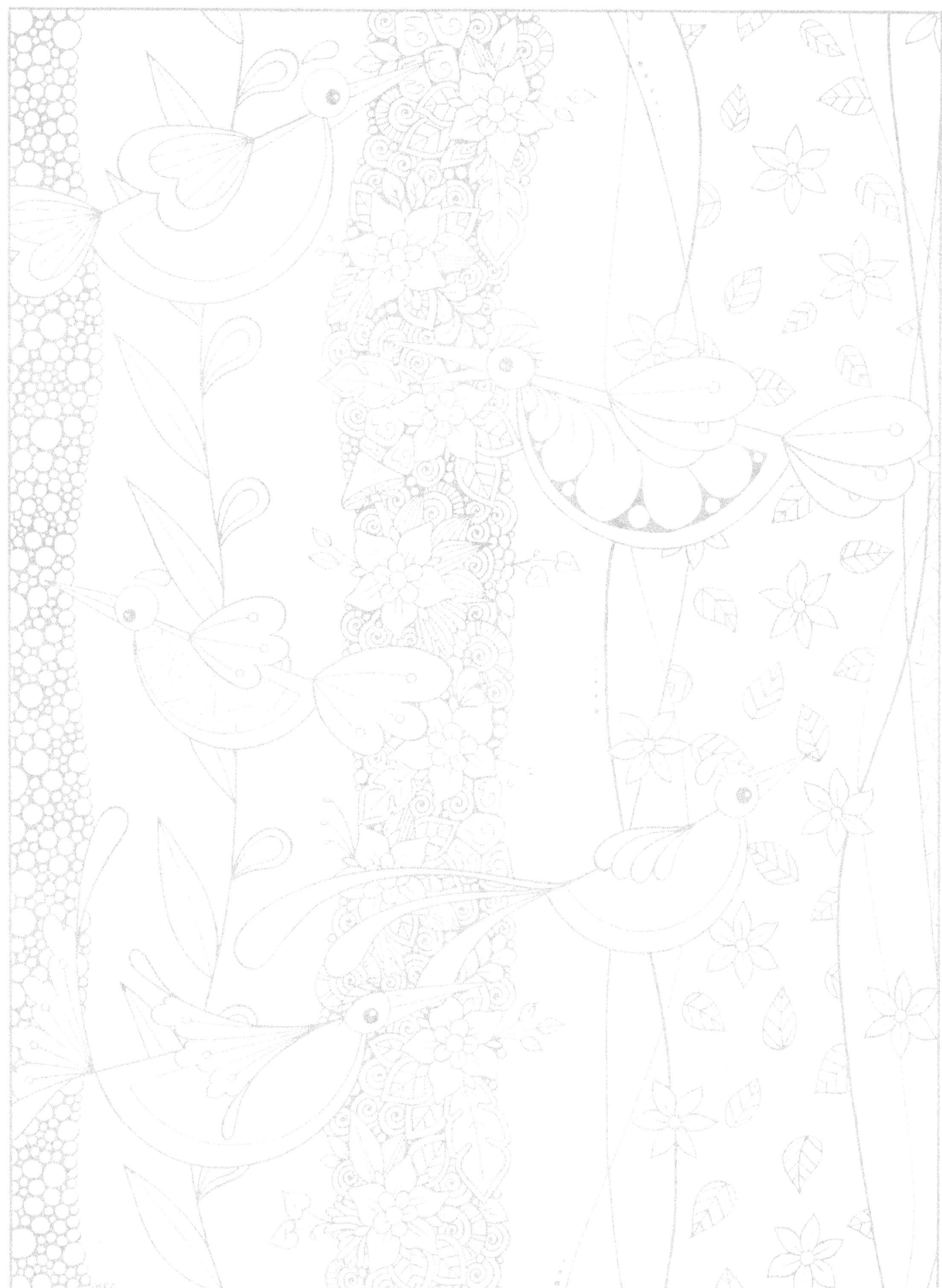

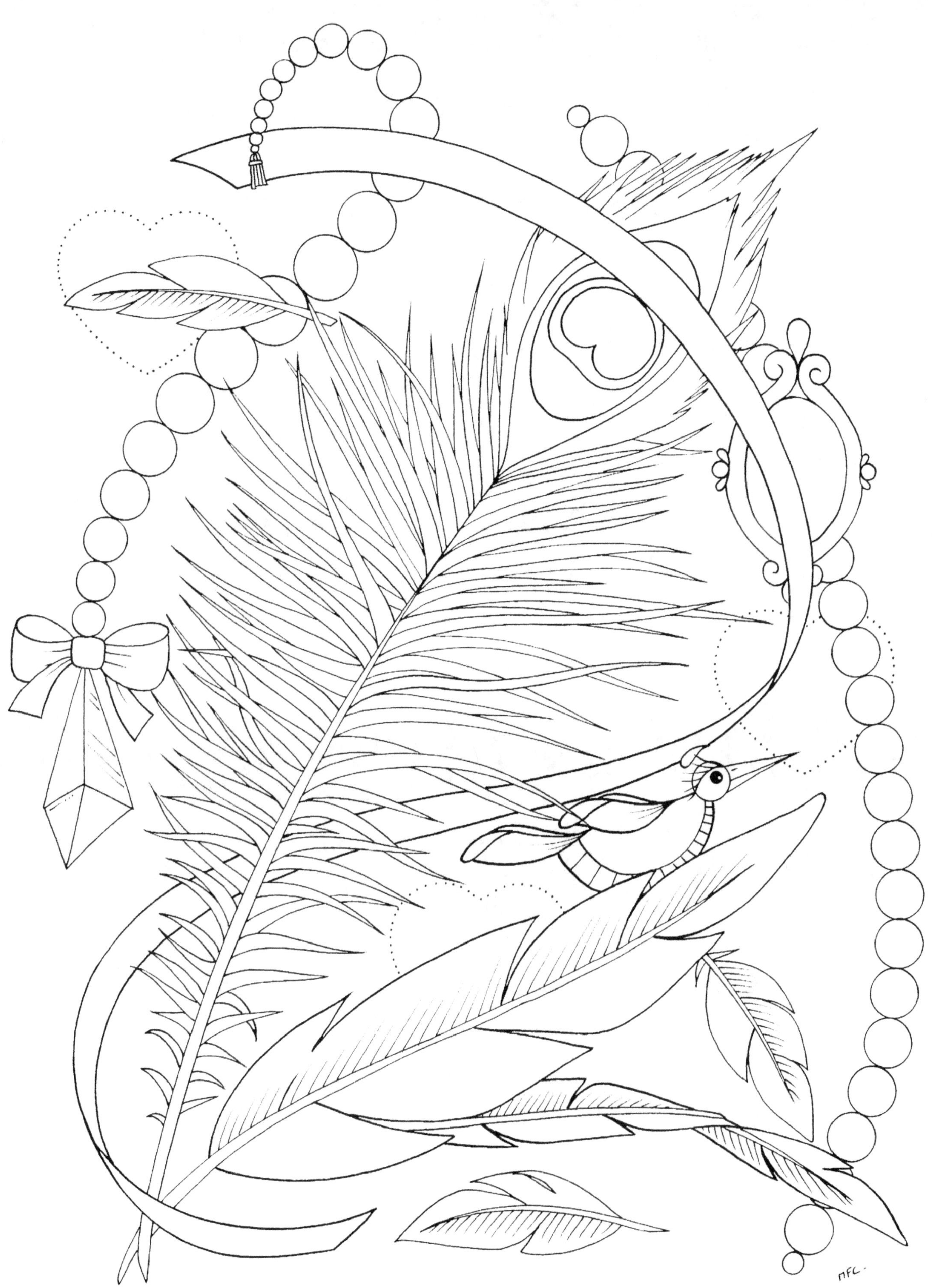

MFL.

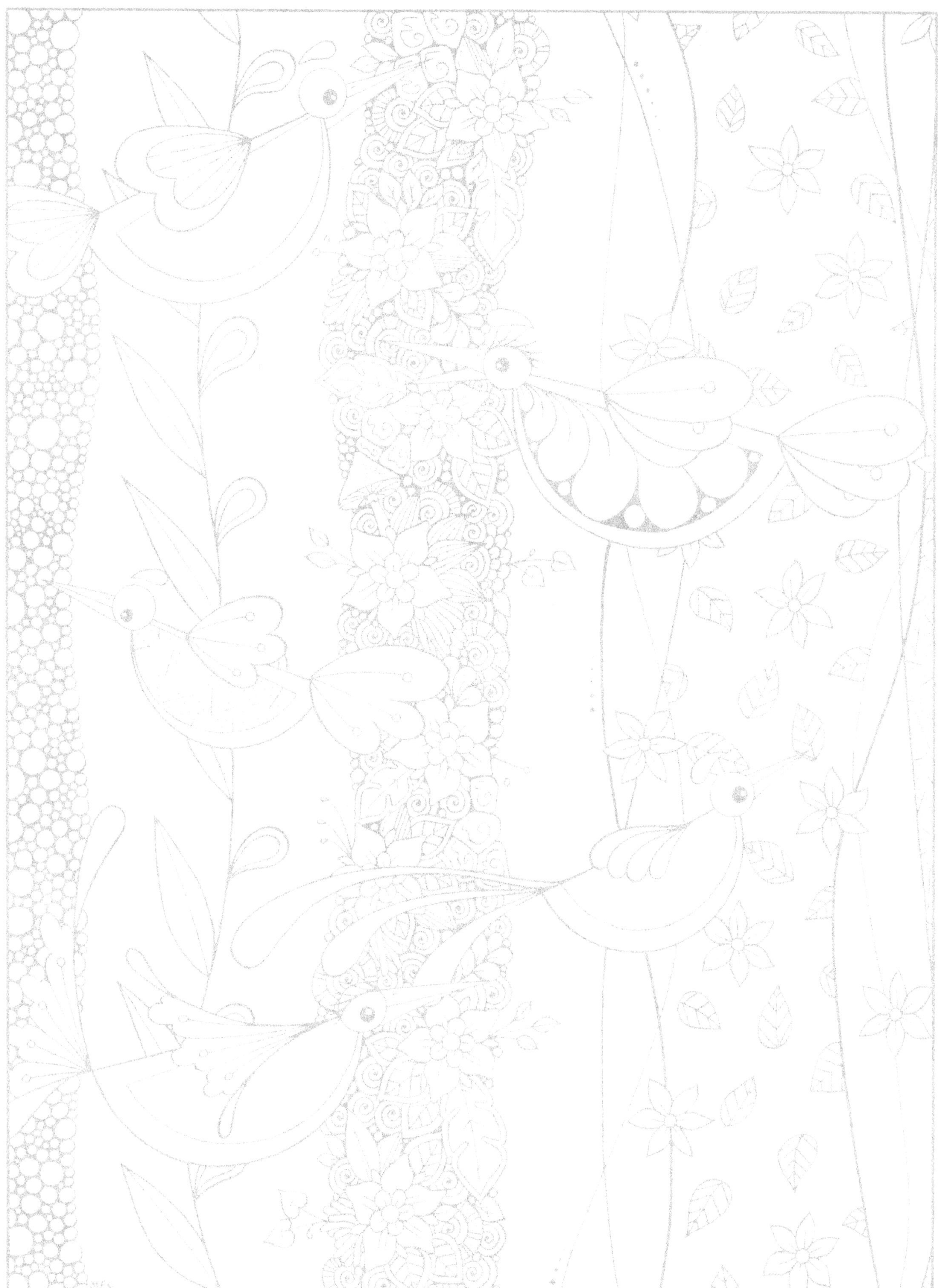

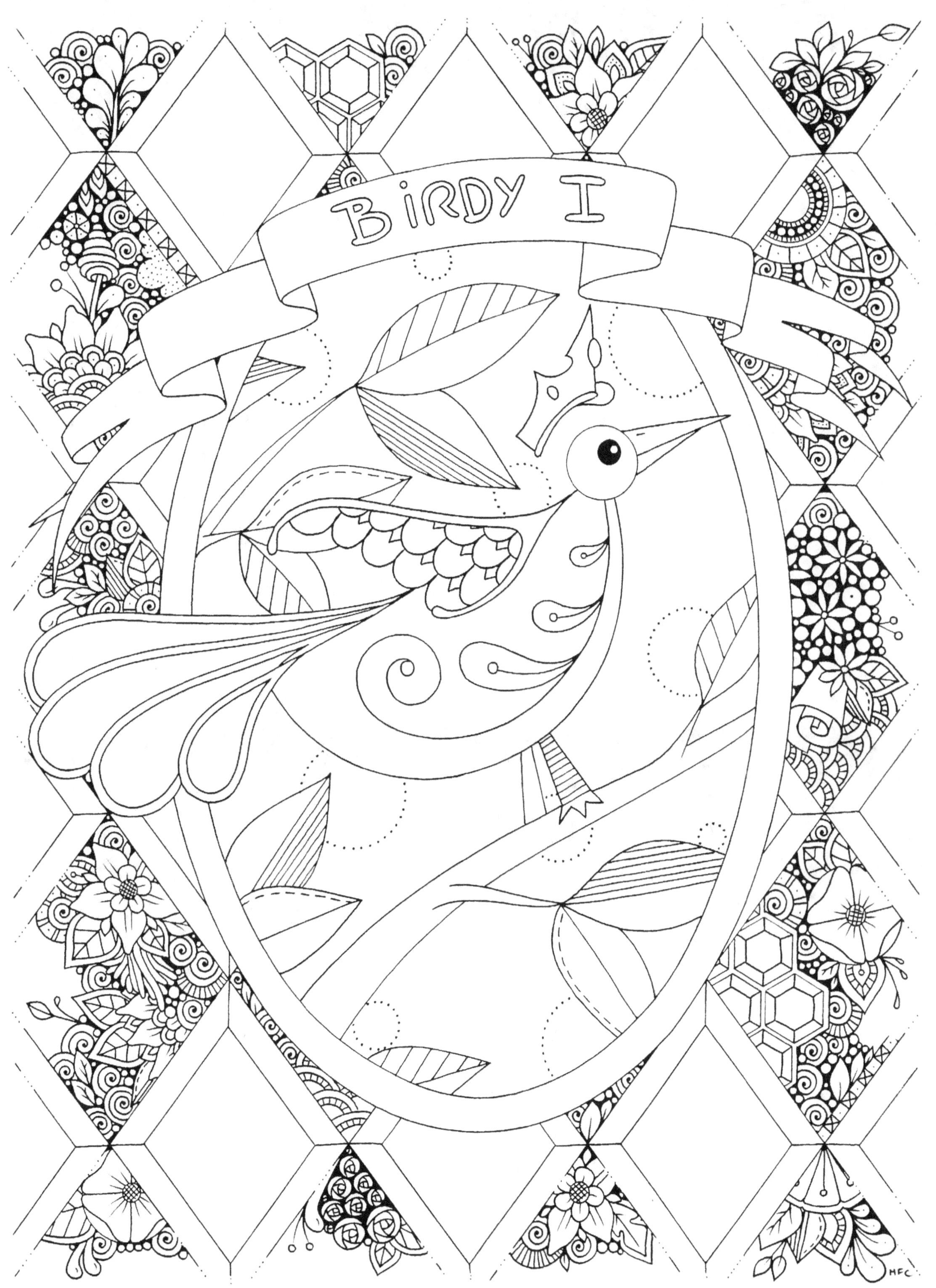
BiRDY I

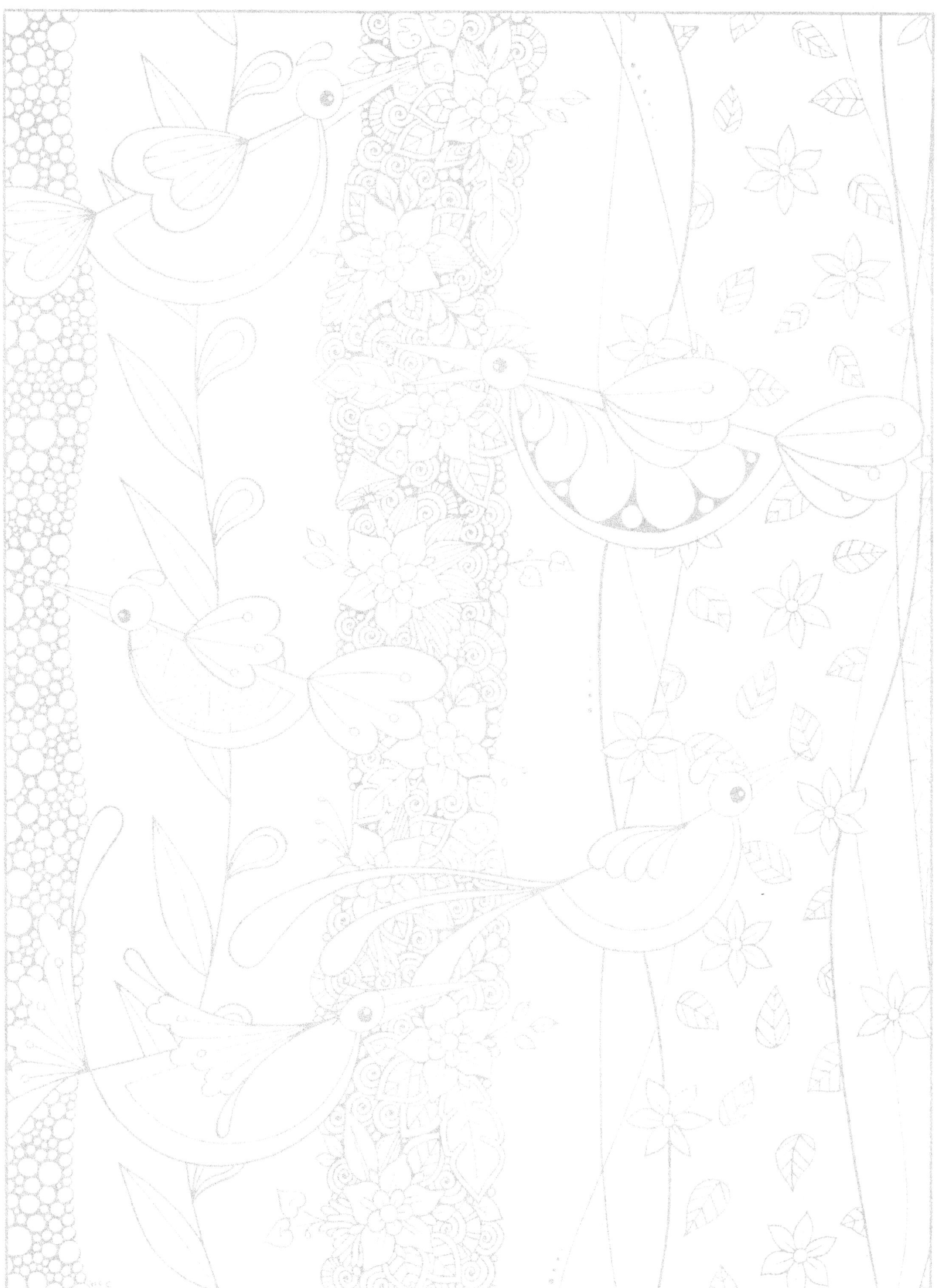

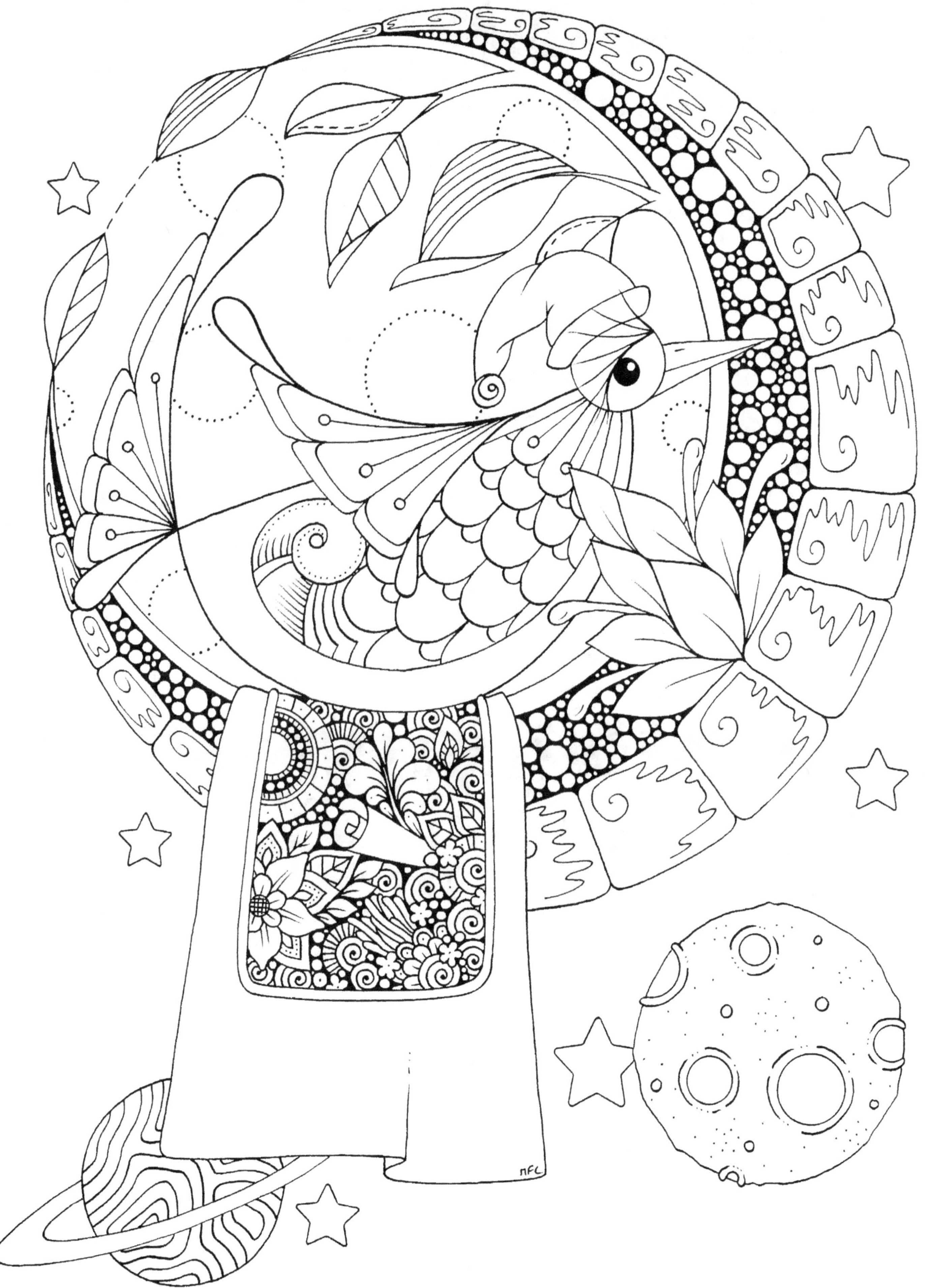

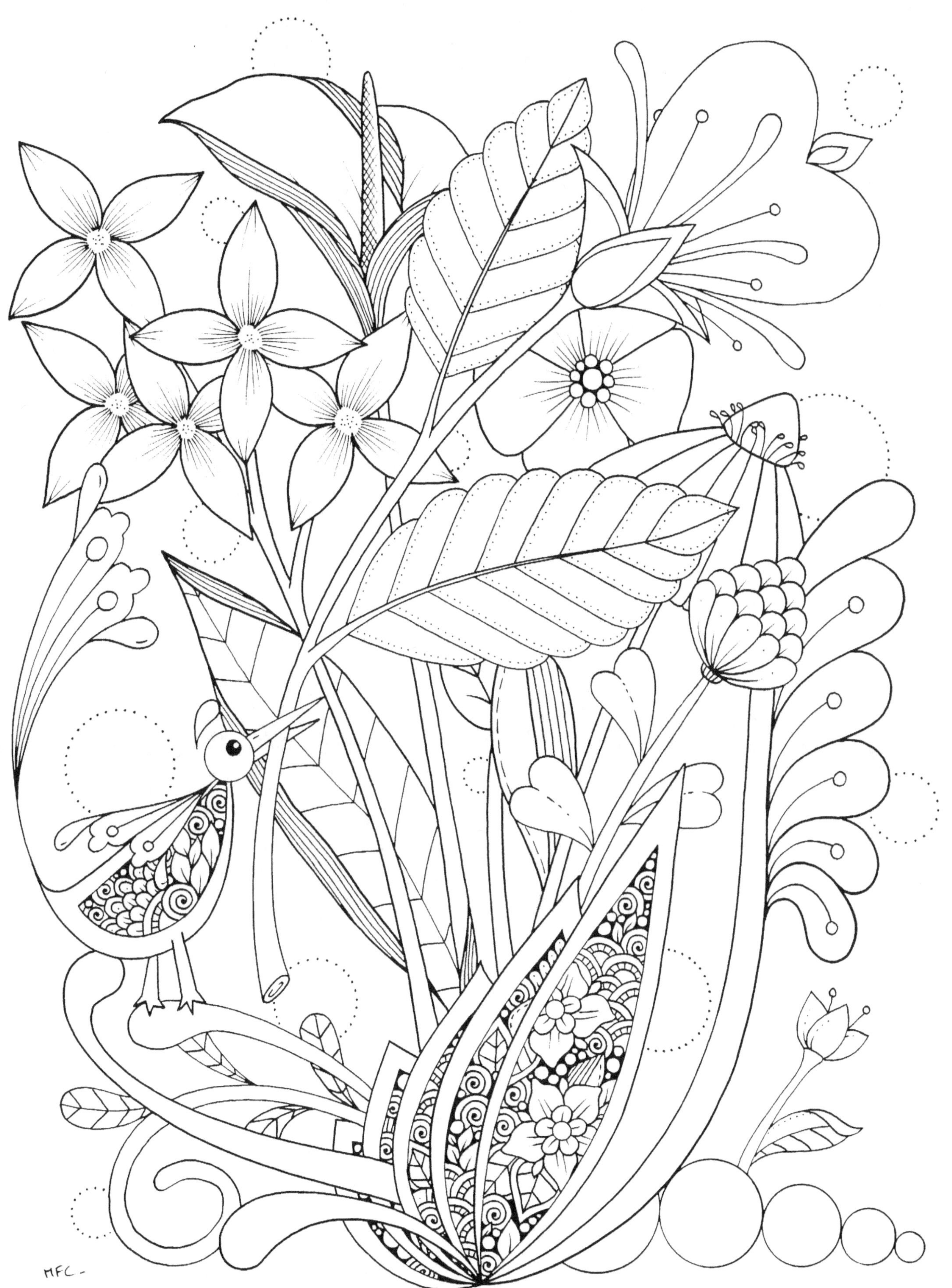
MFC

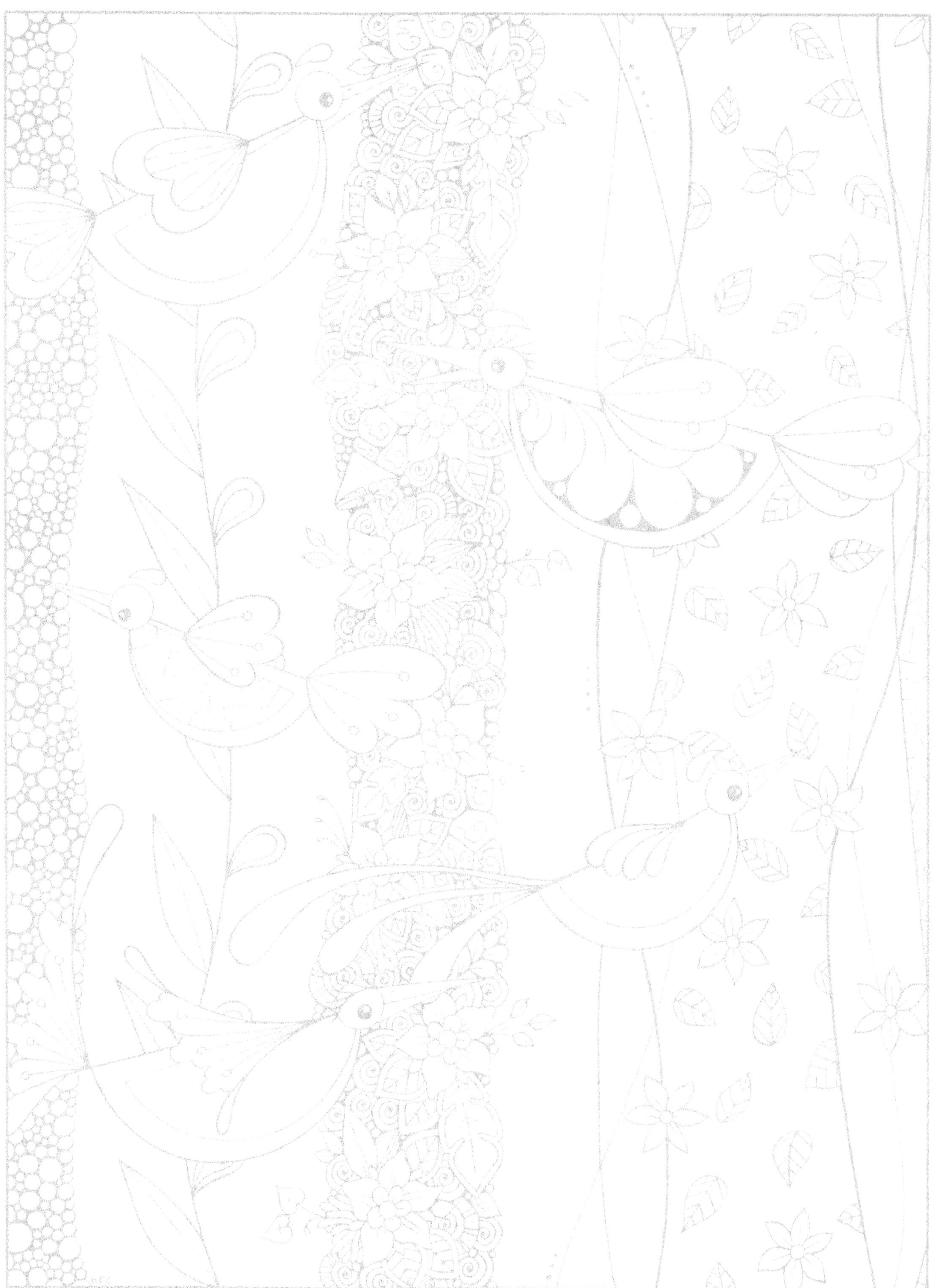

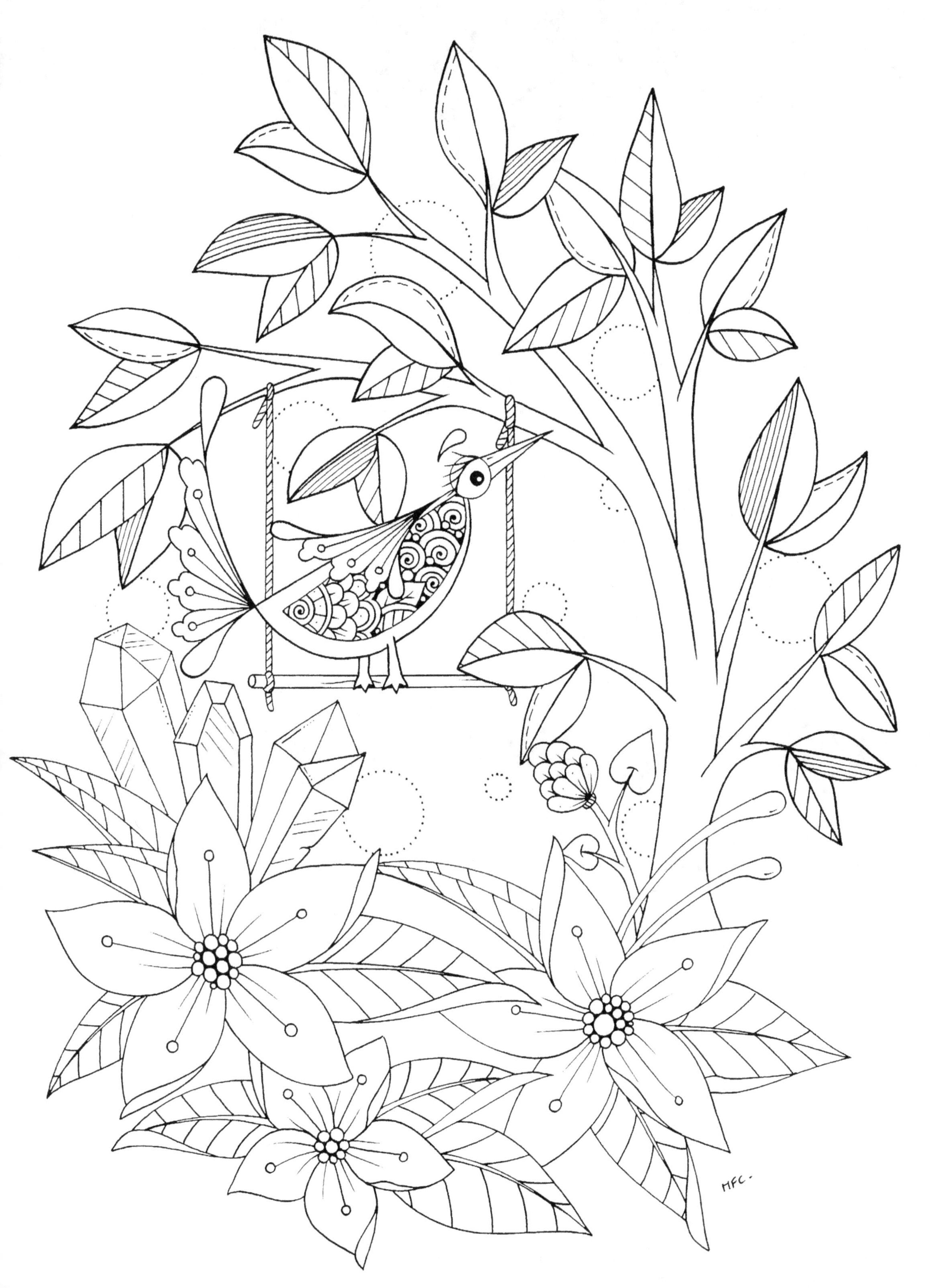

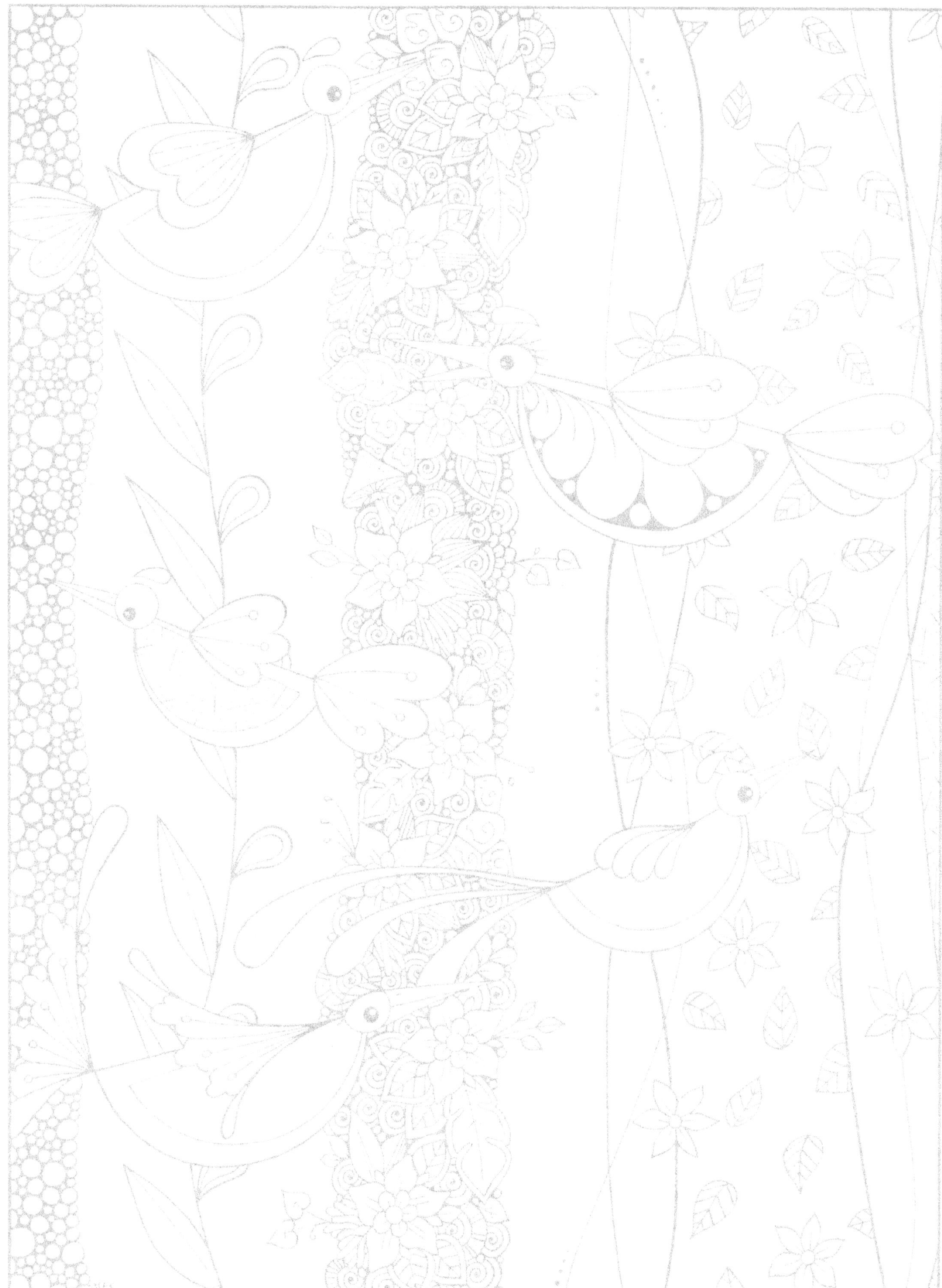

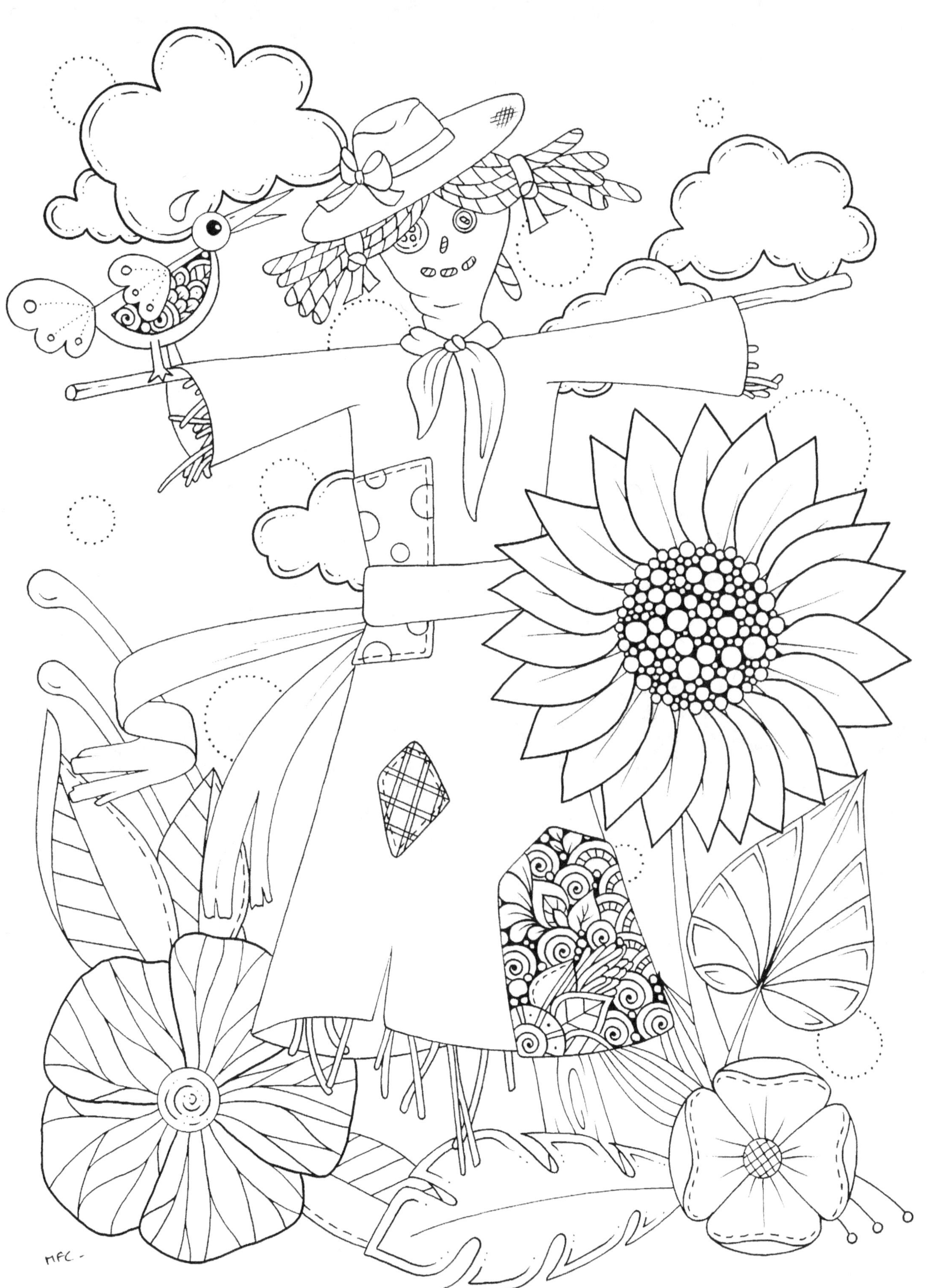

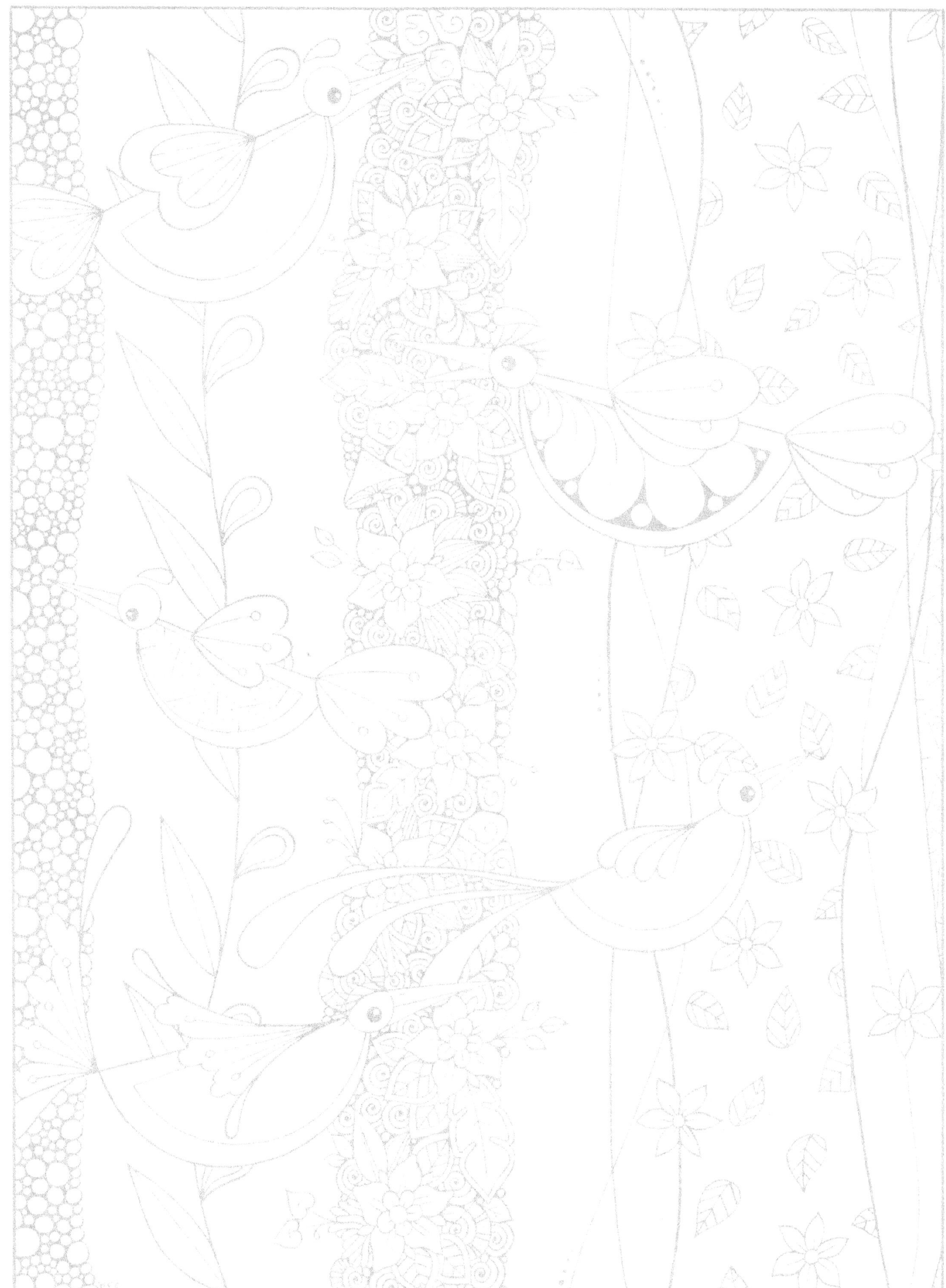

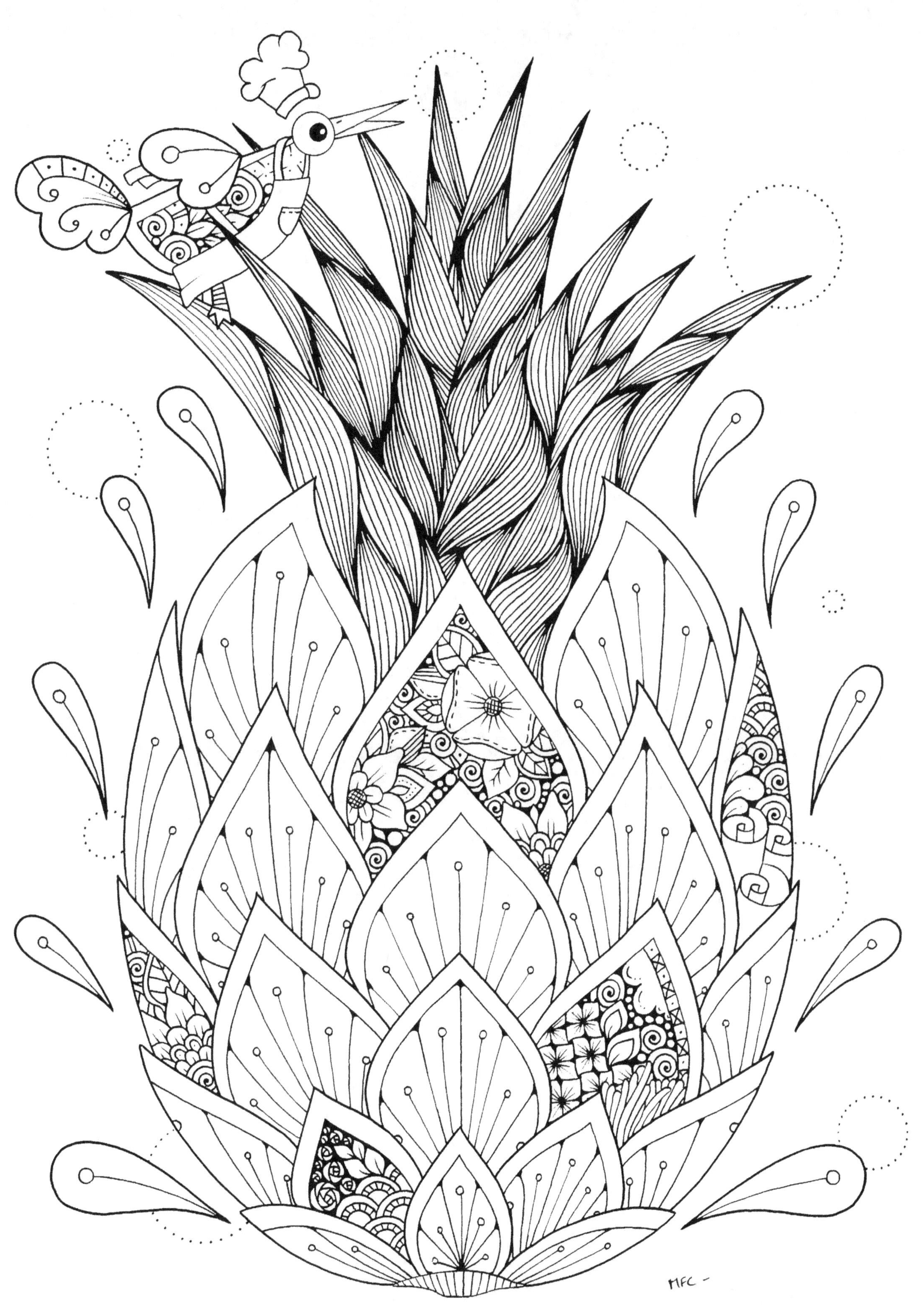

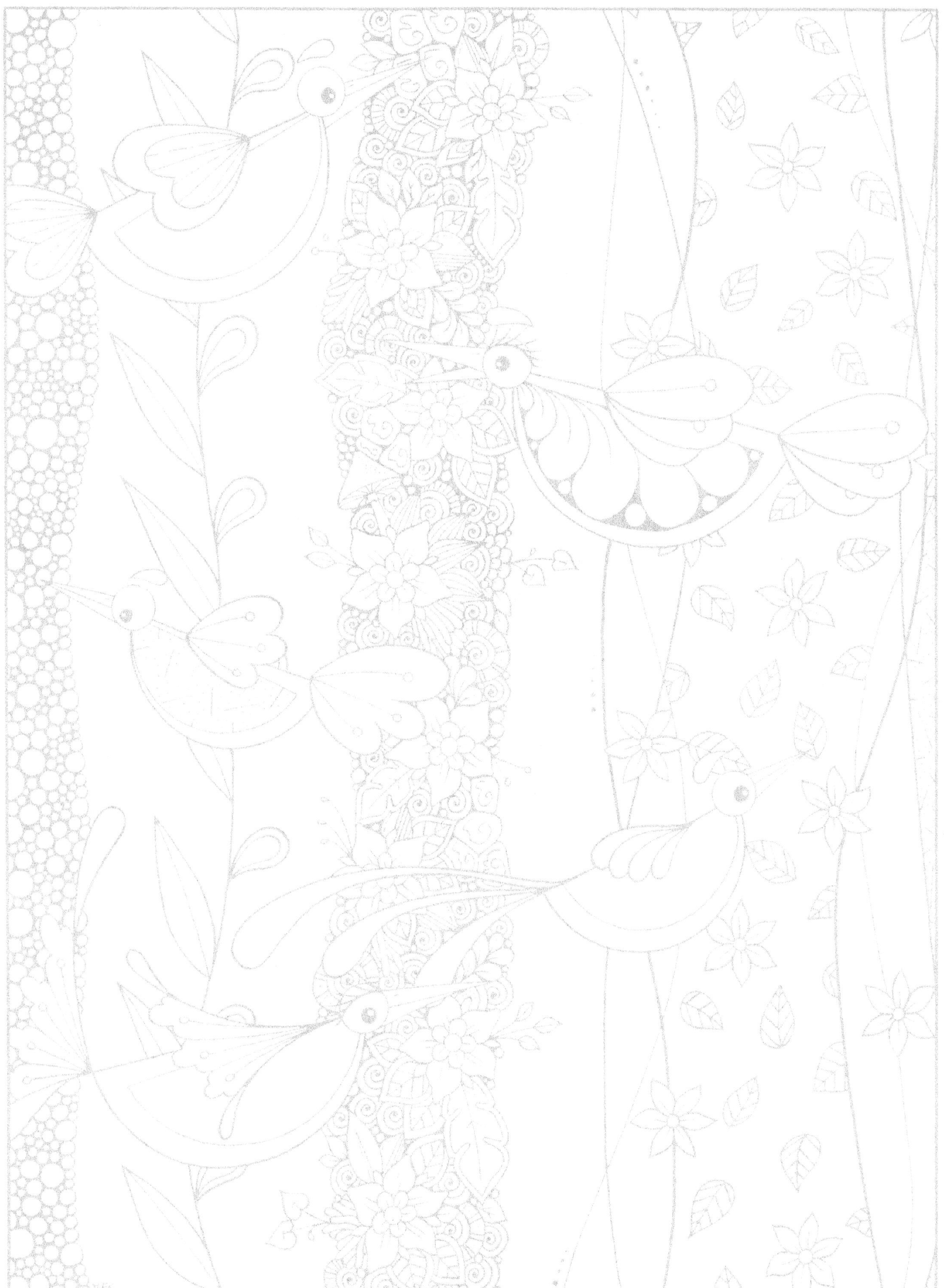

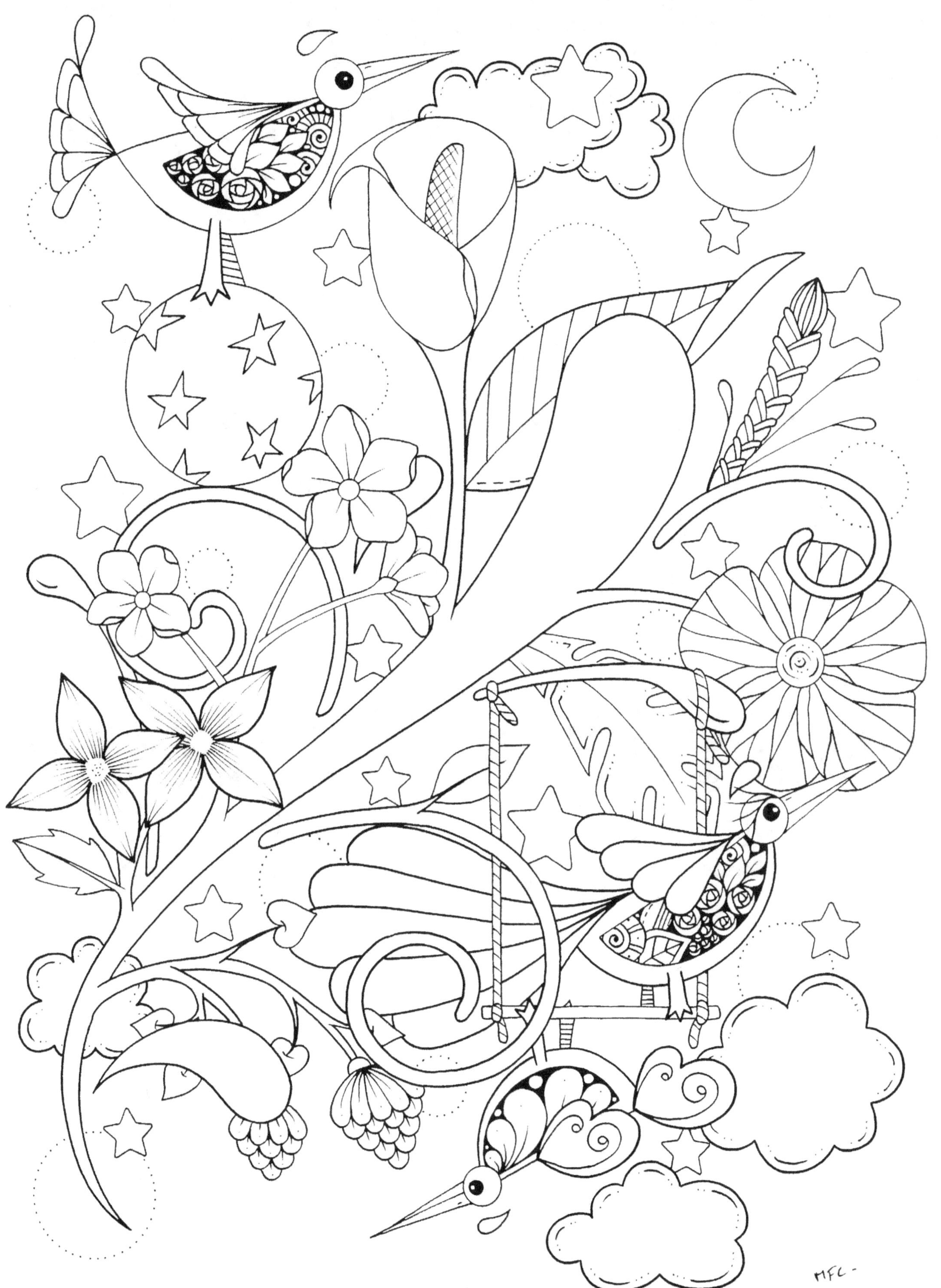

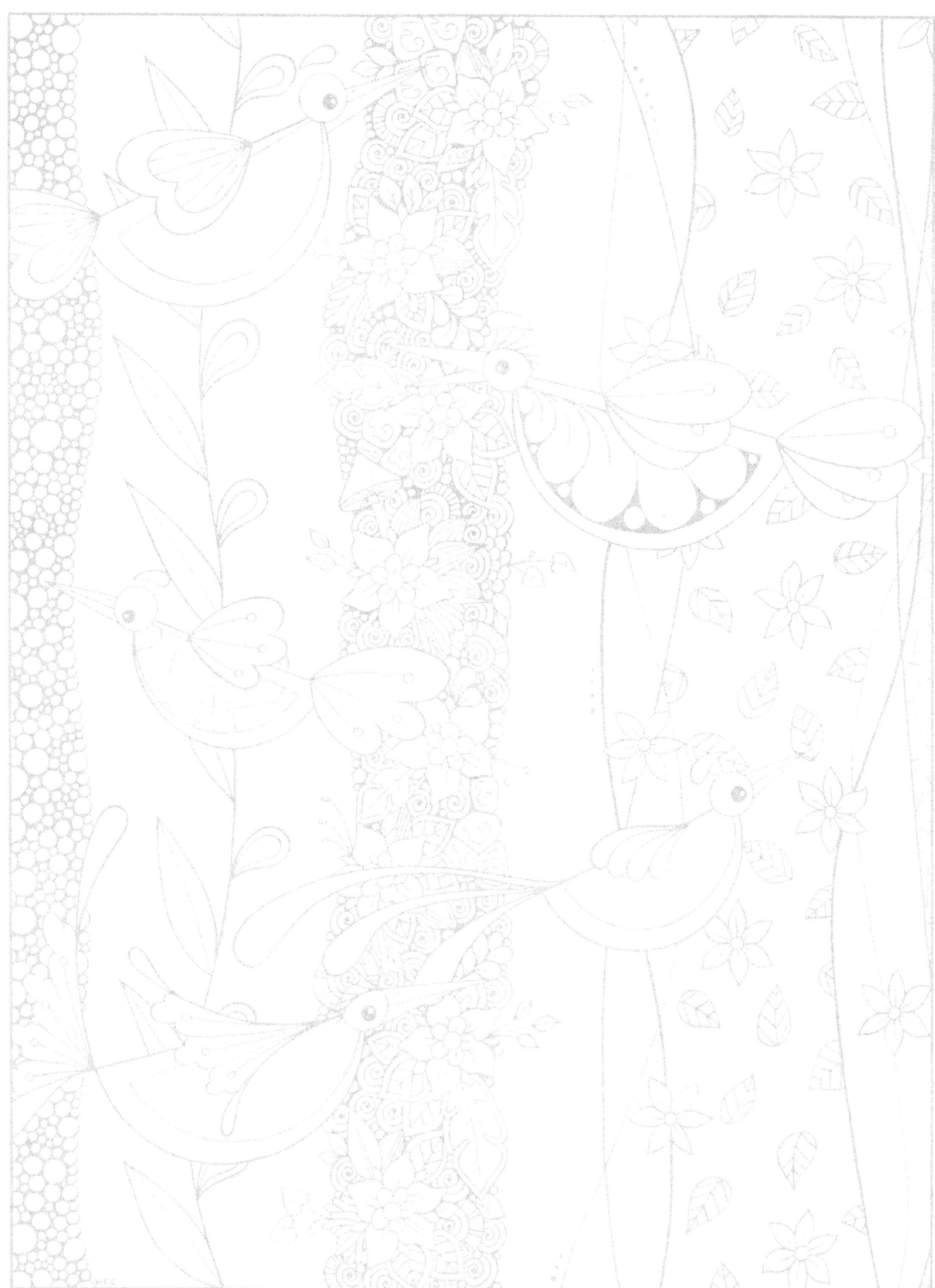

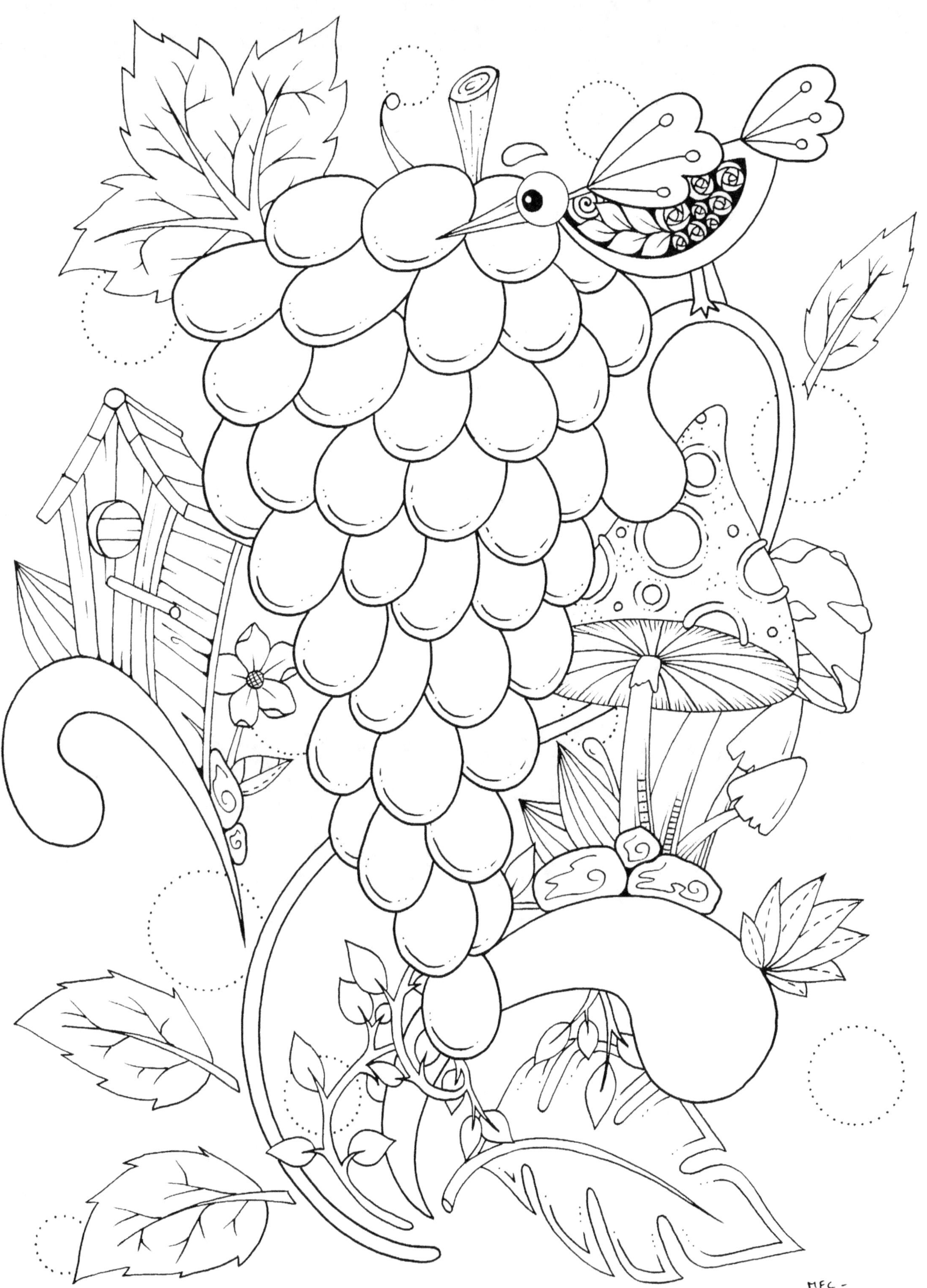

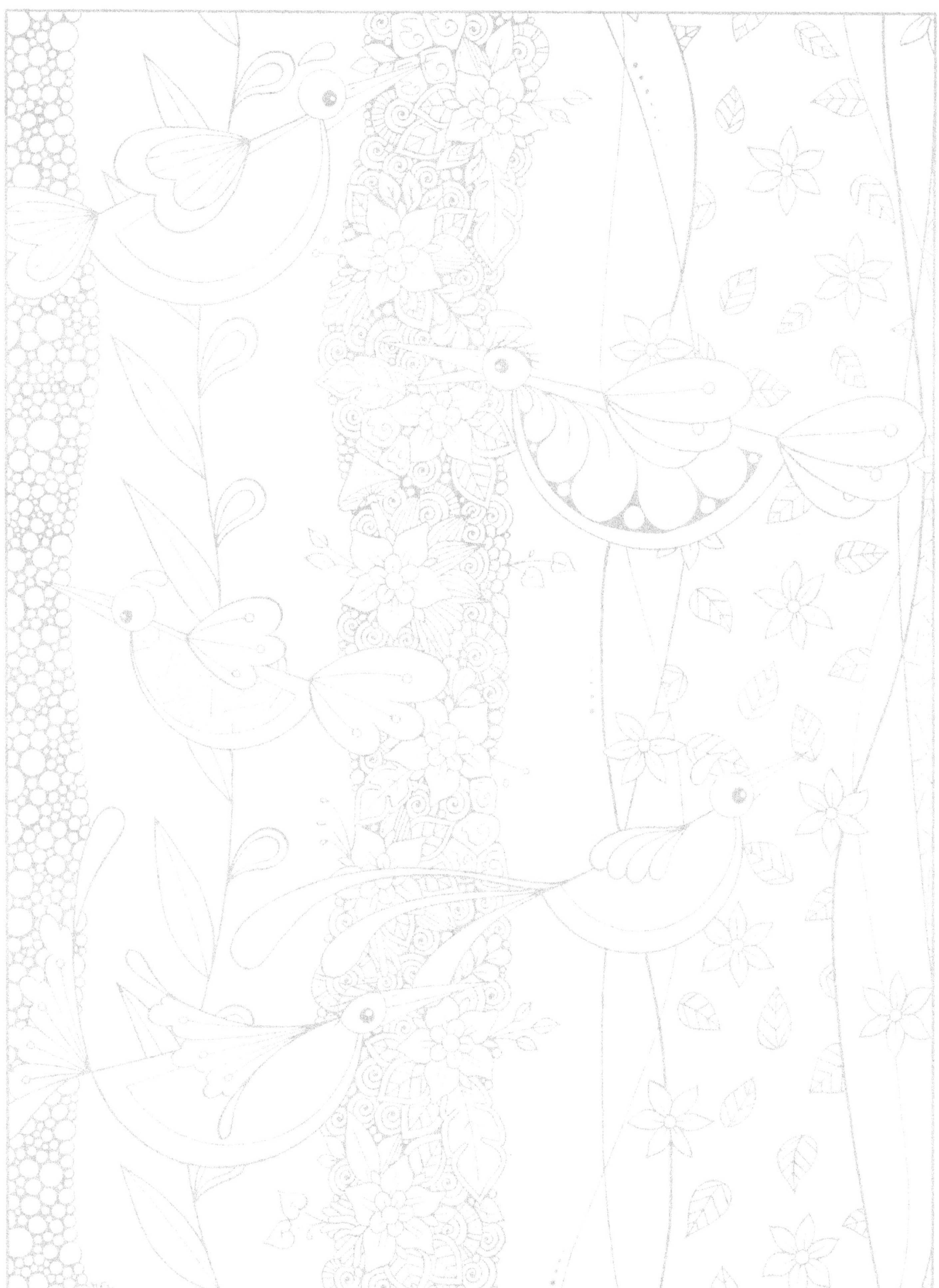

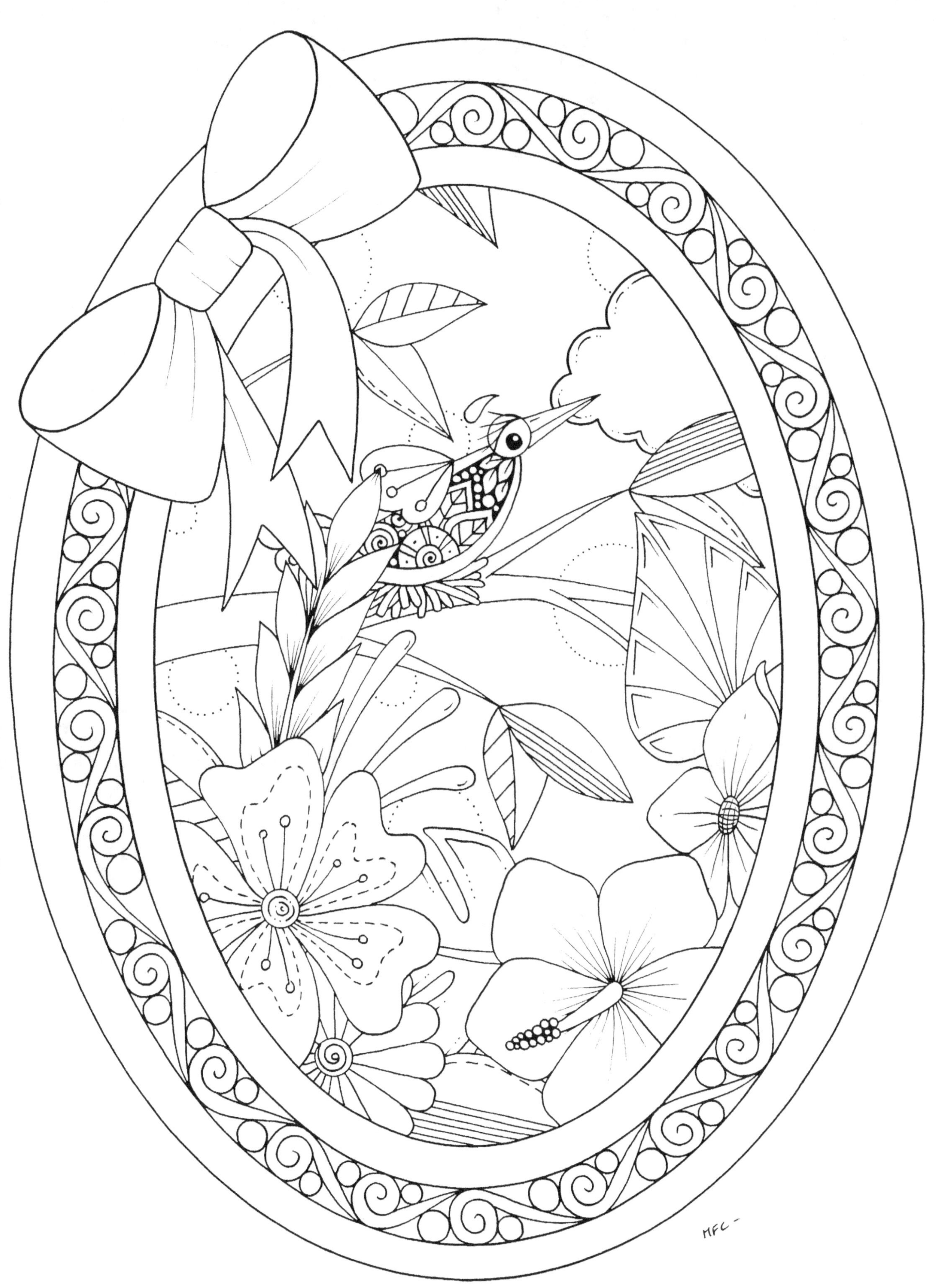

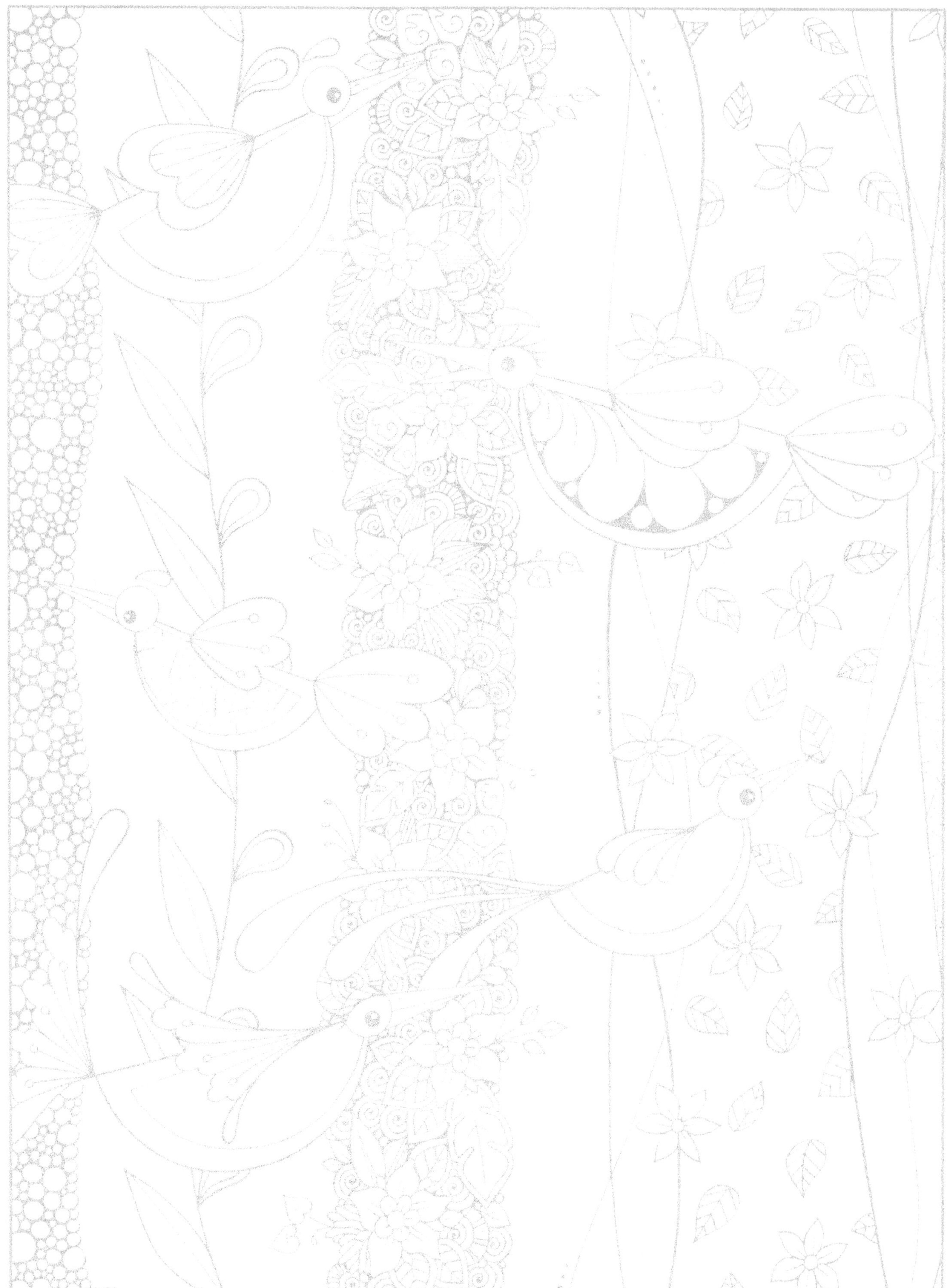

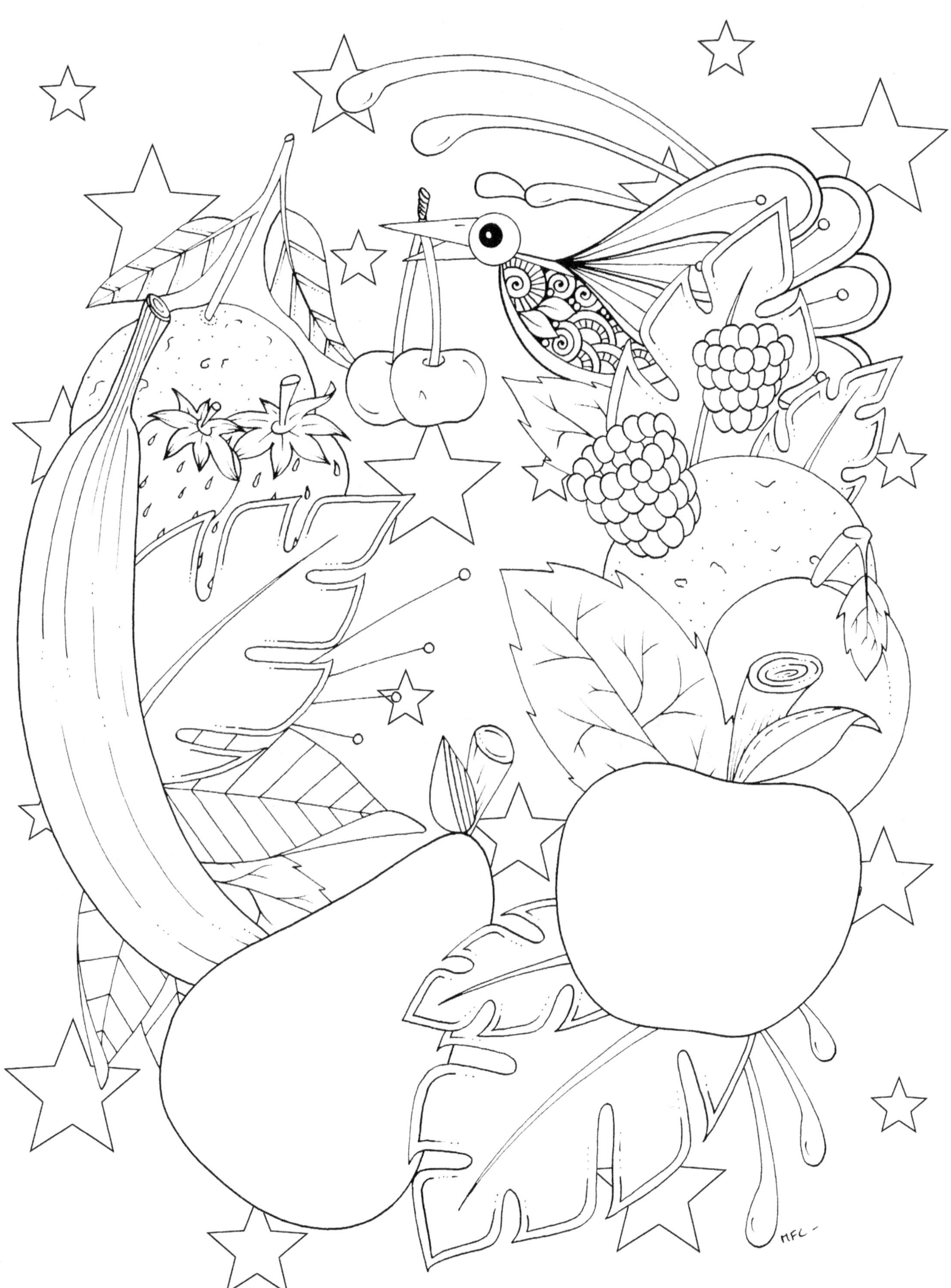

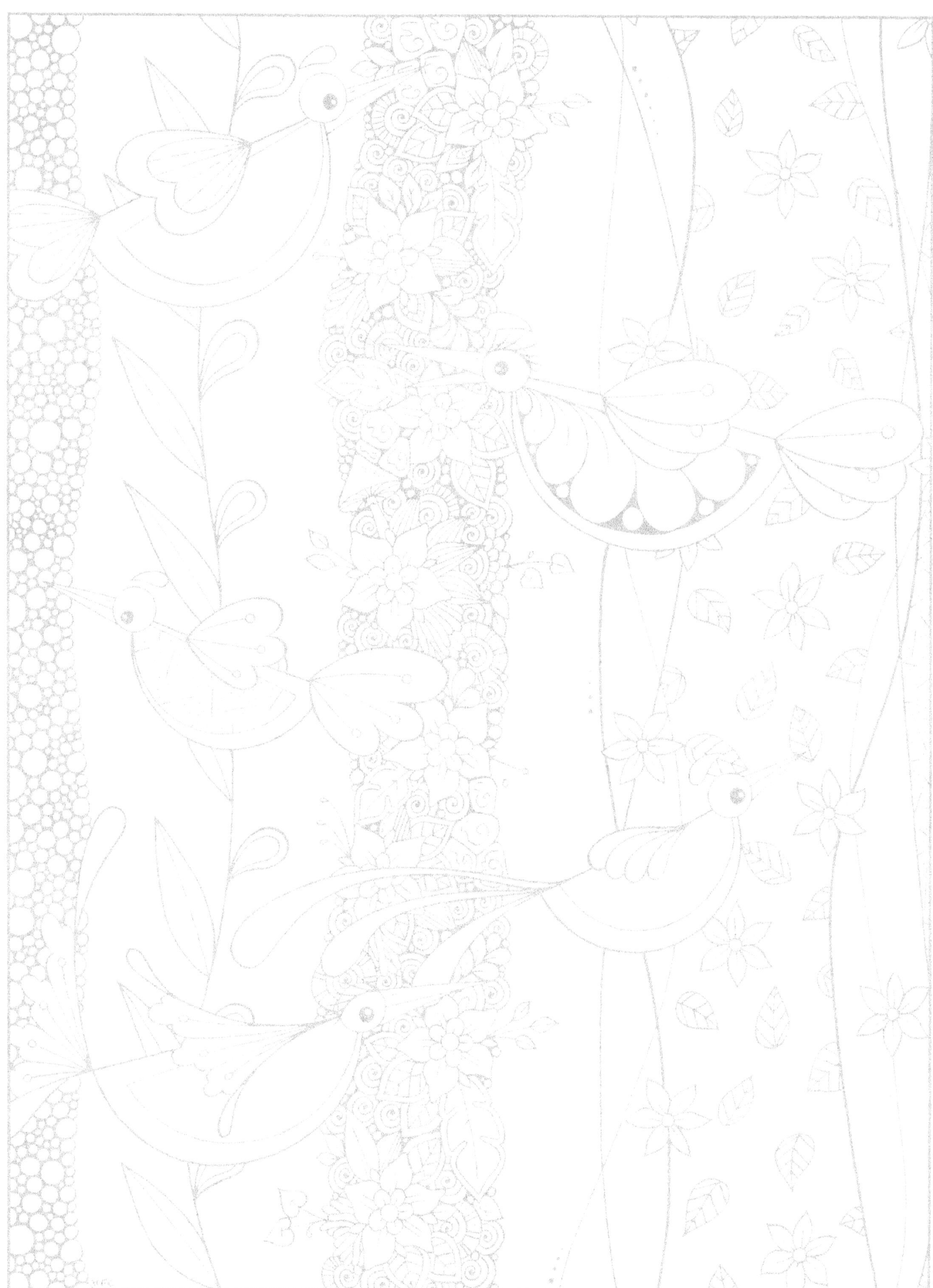

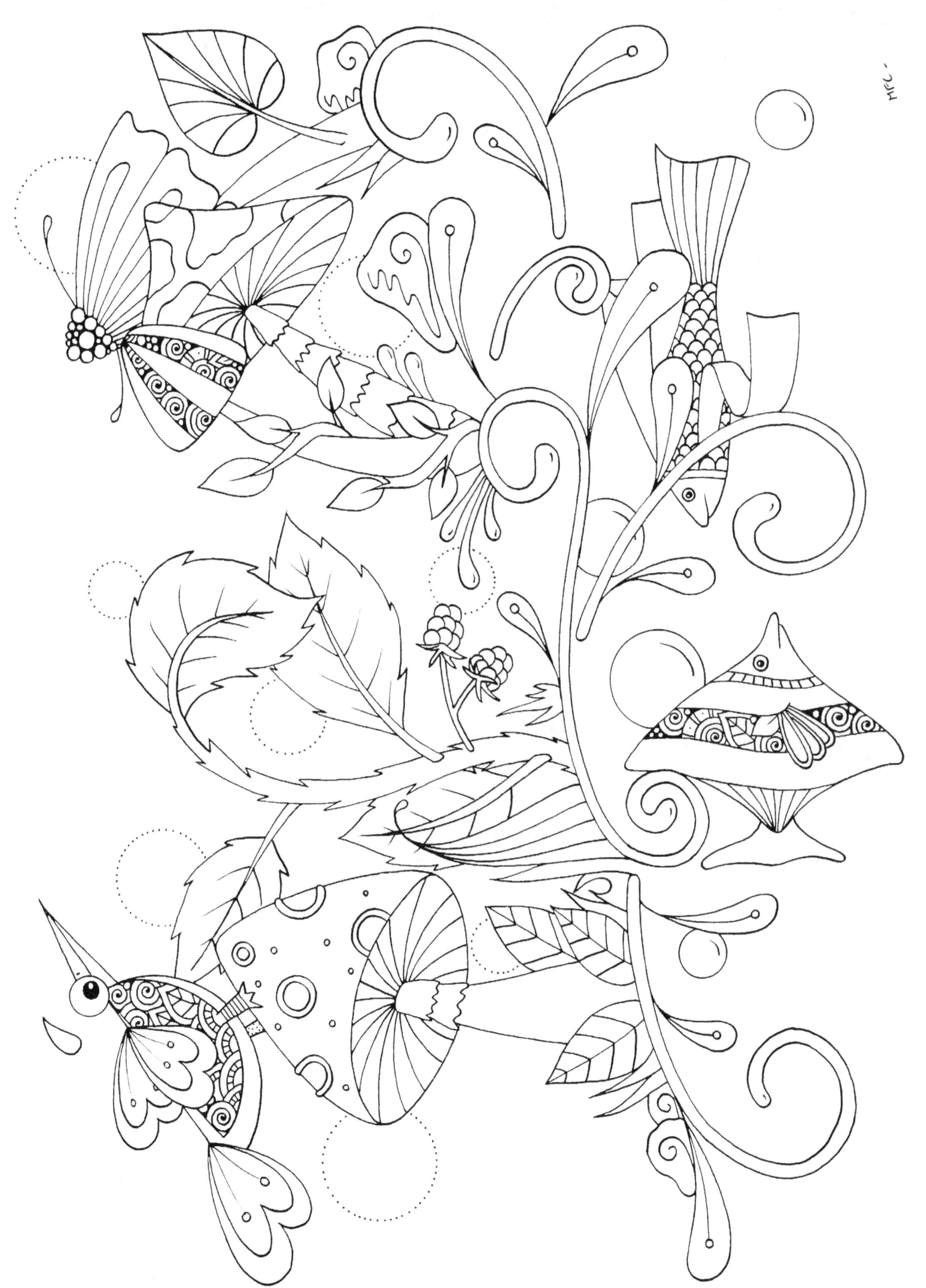

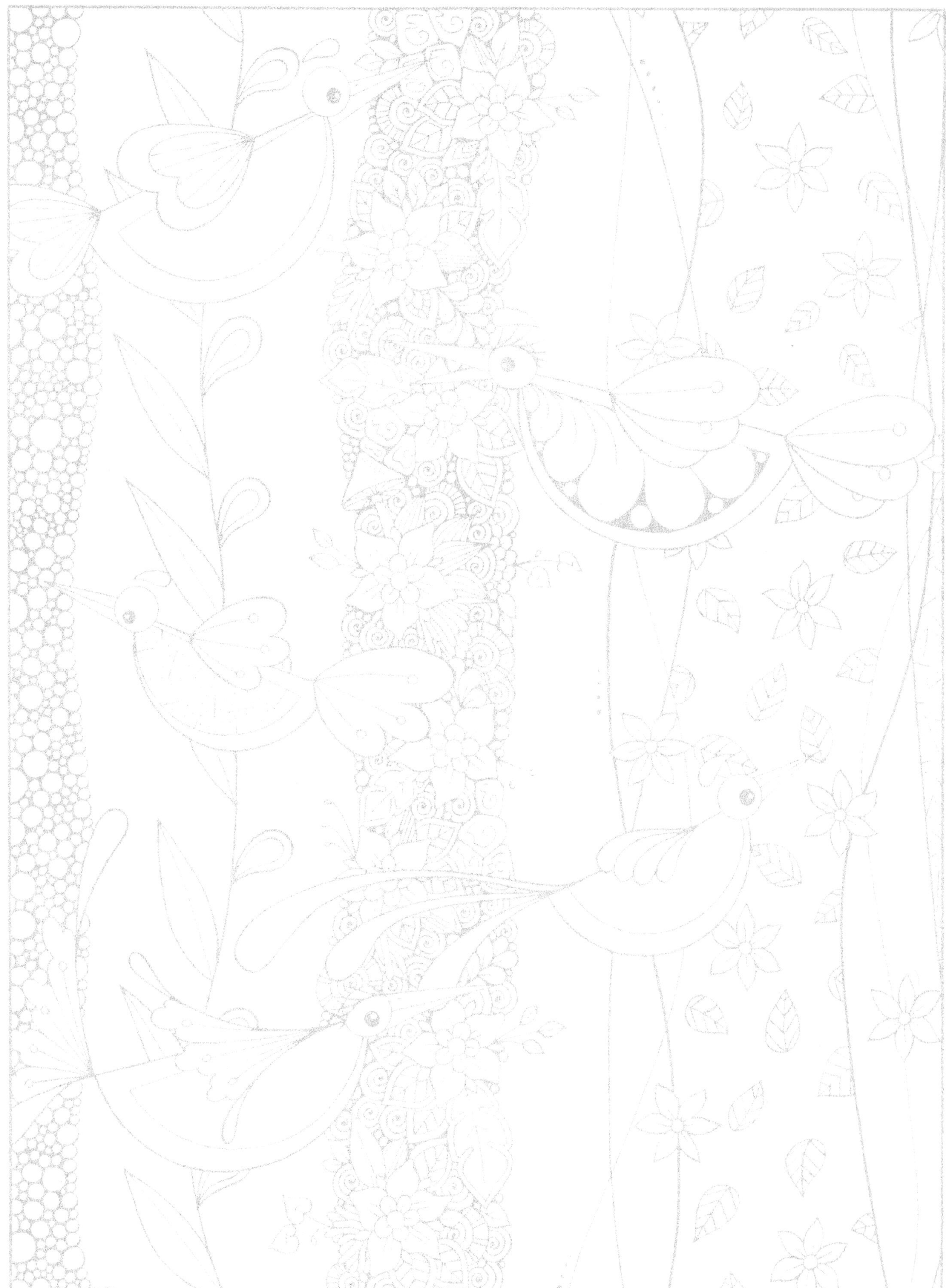

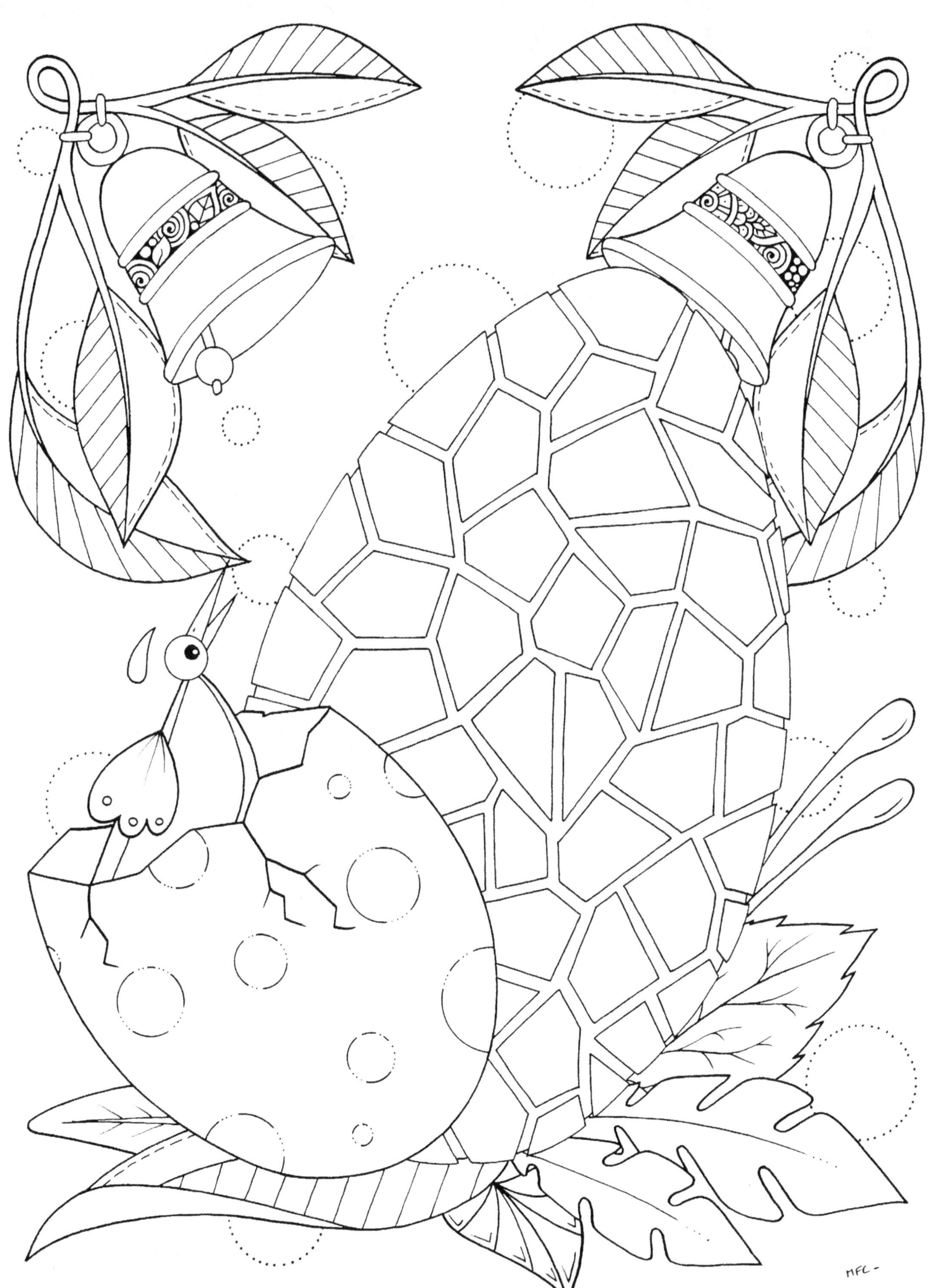

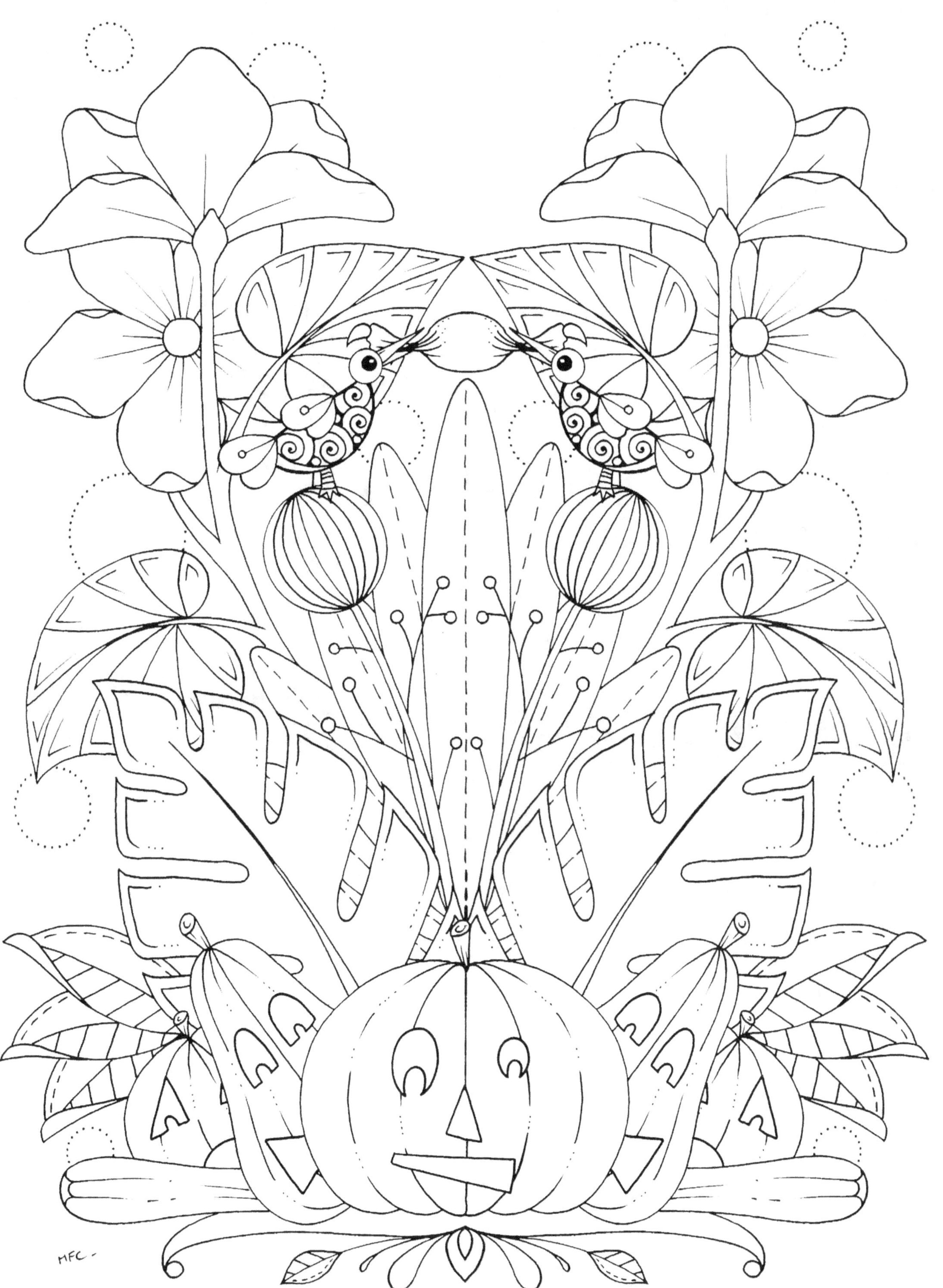

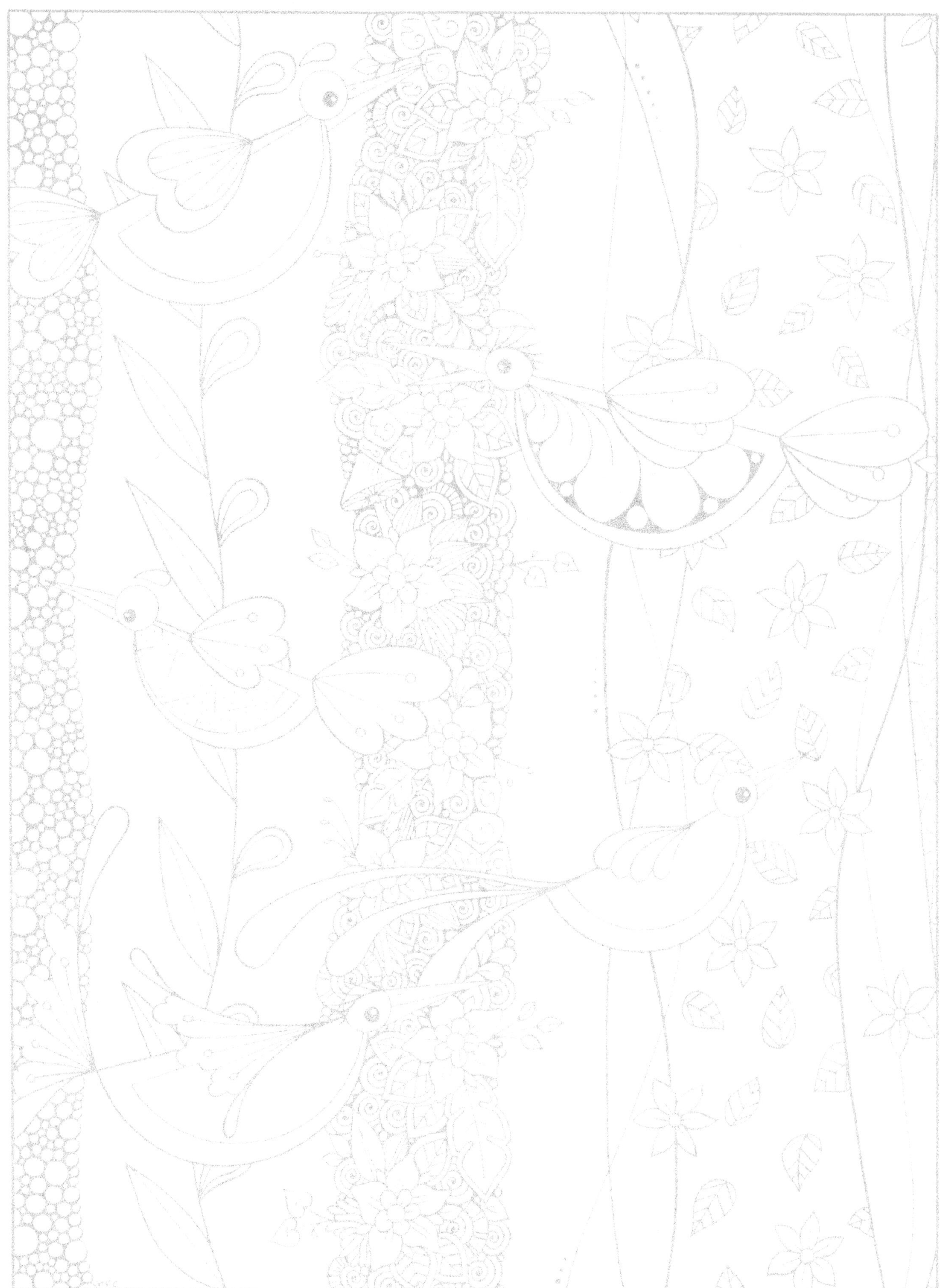

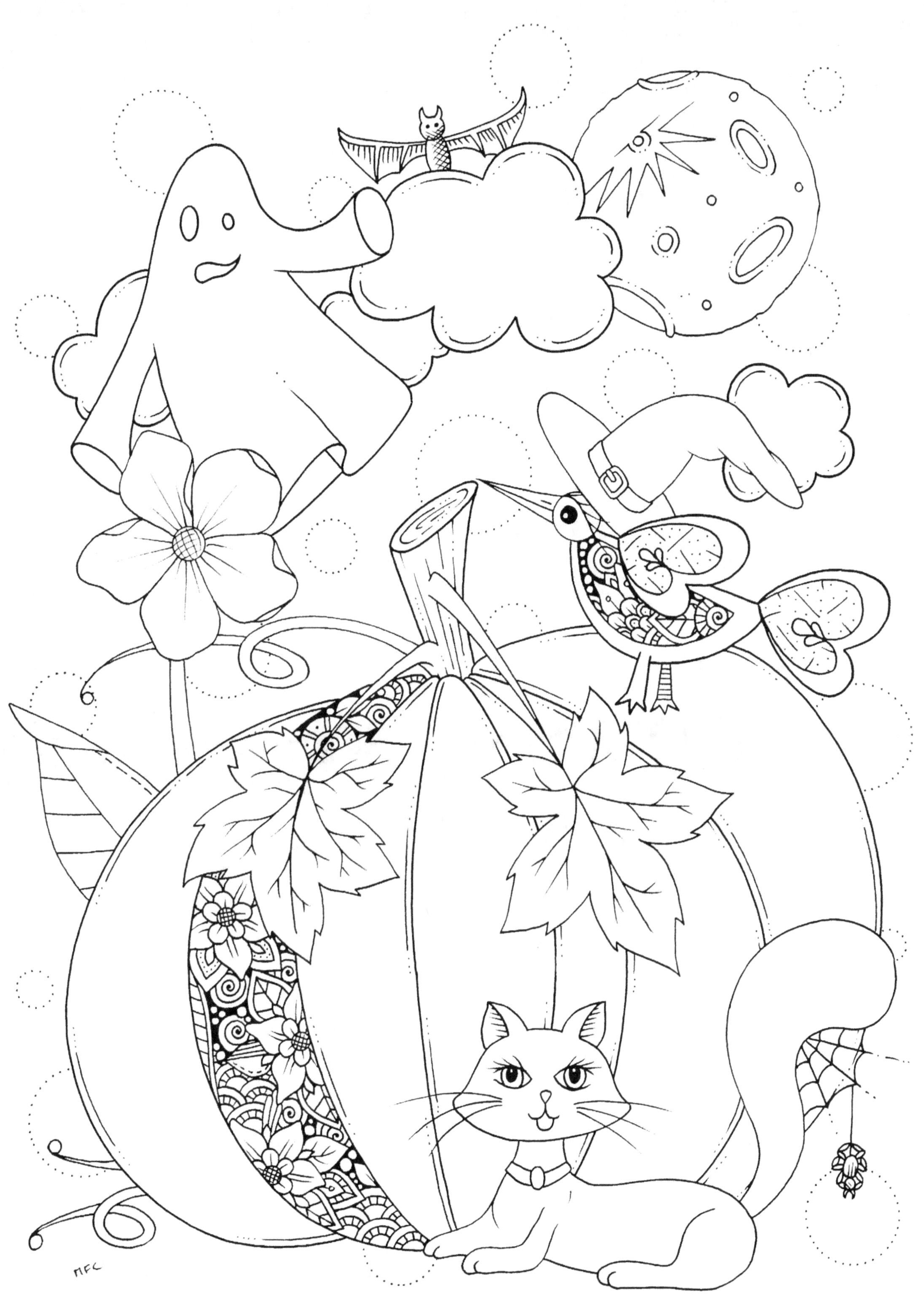

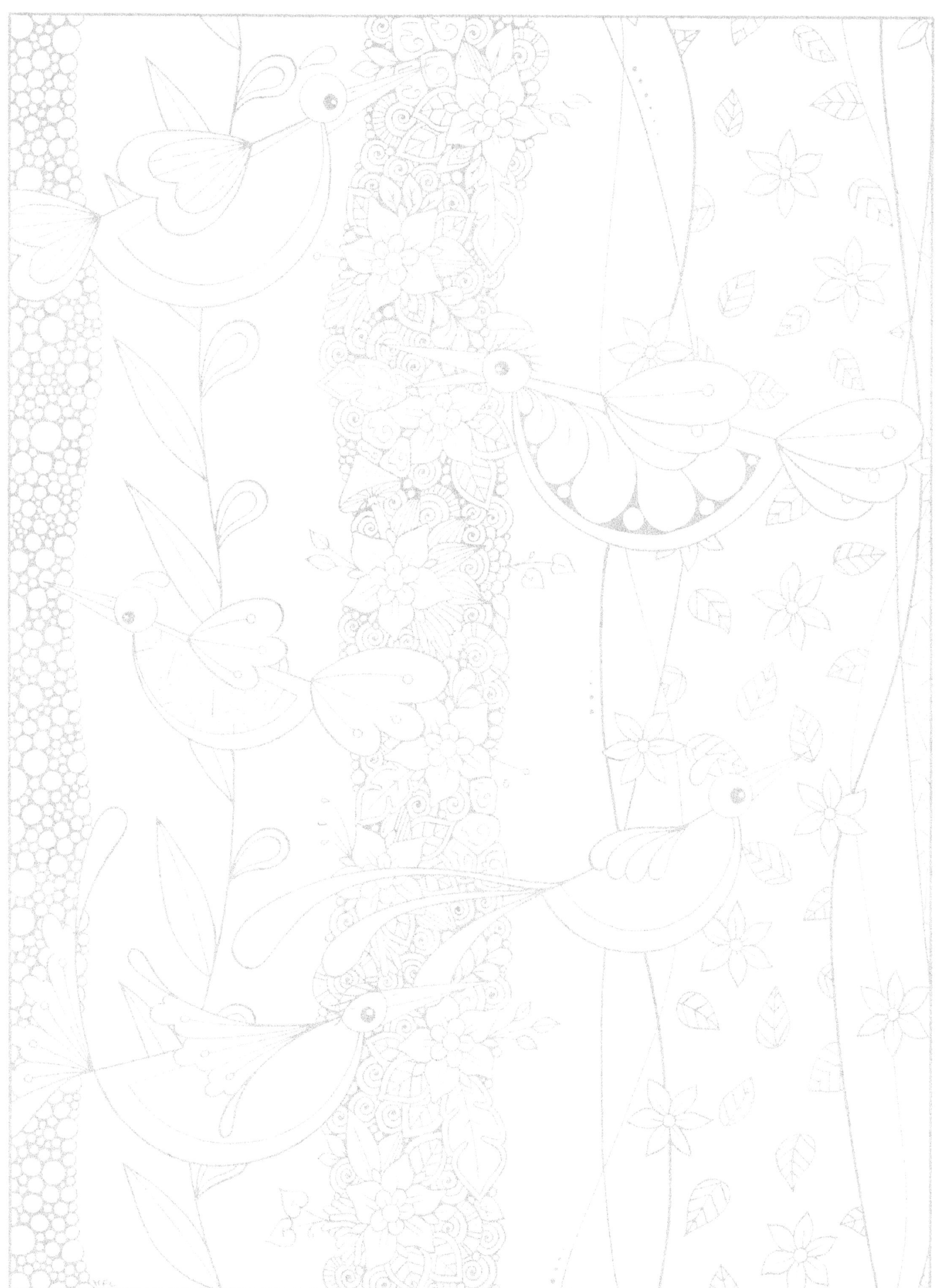

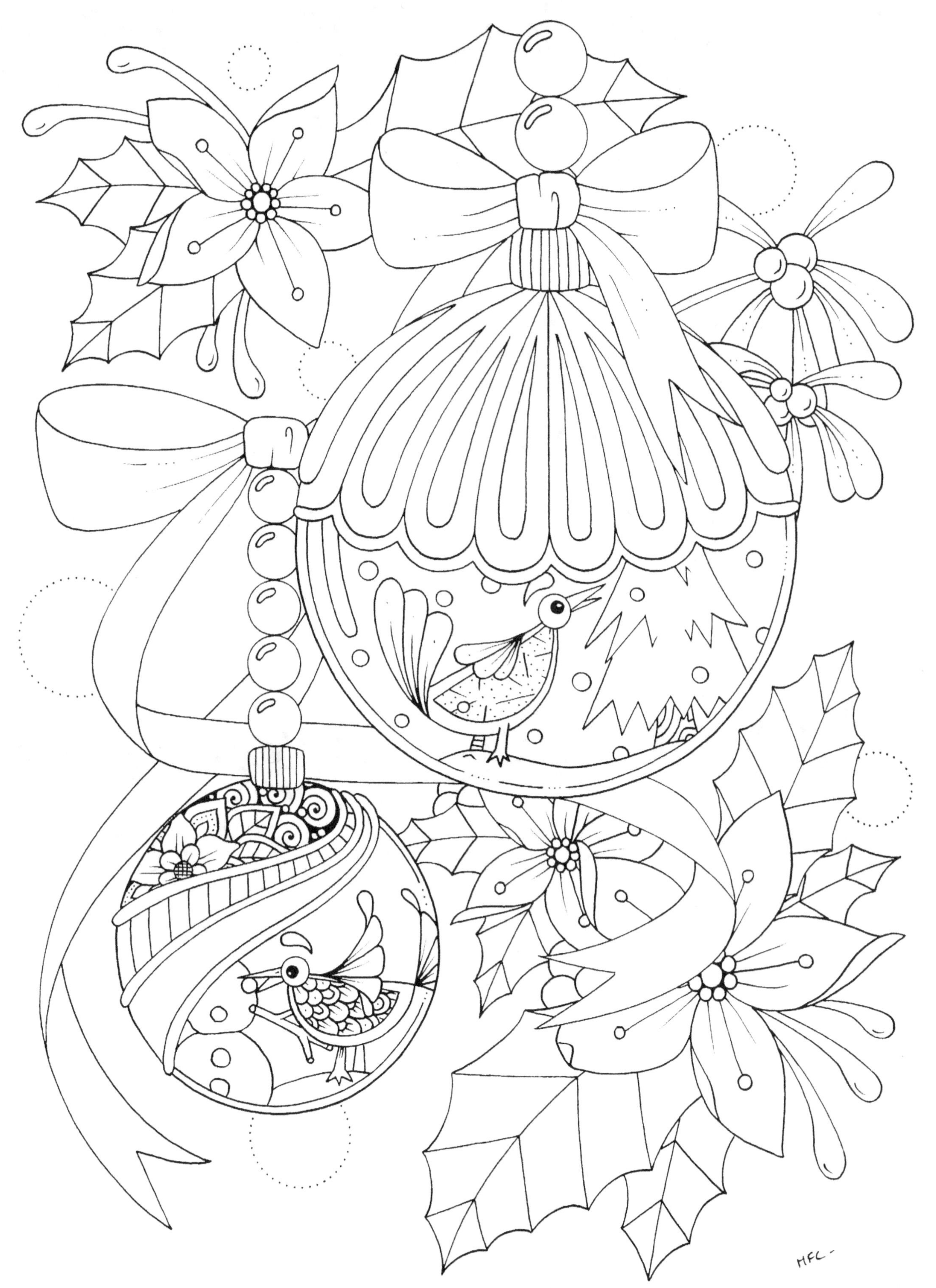
MFC

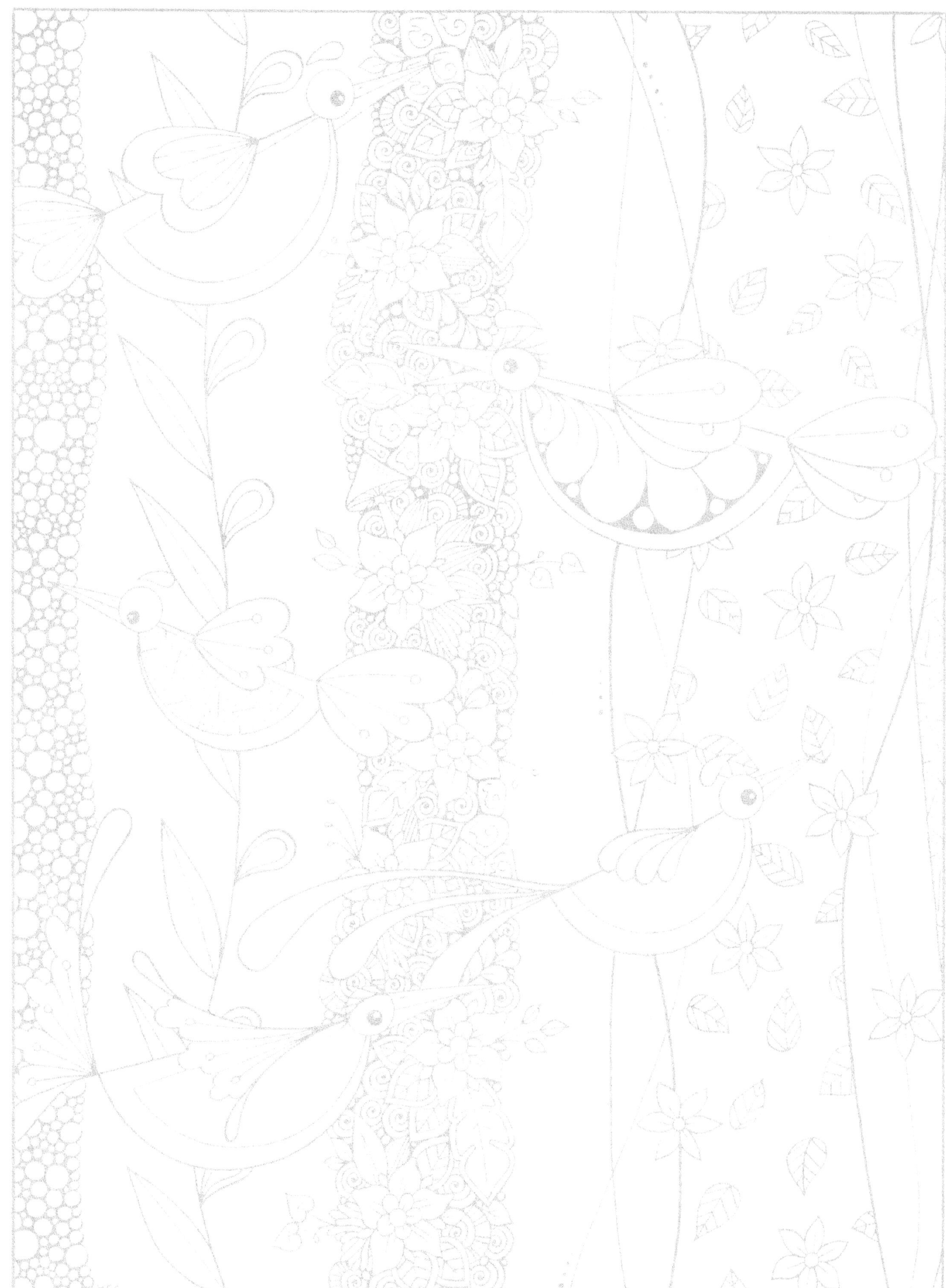

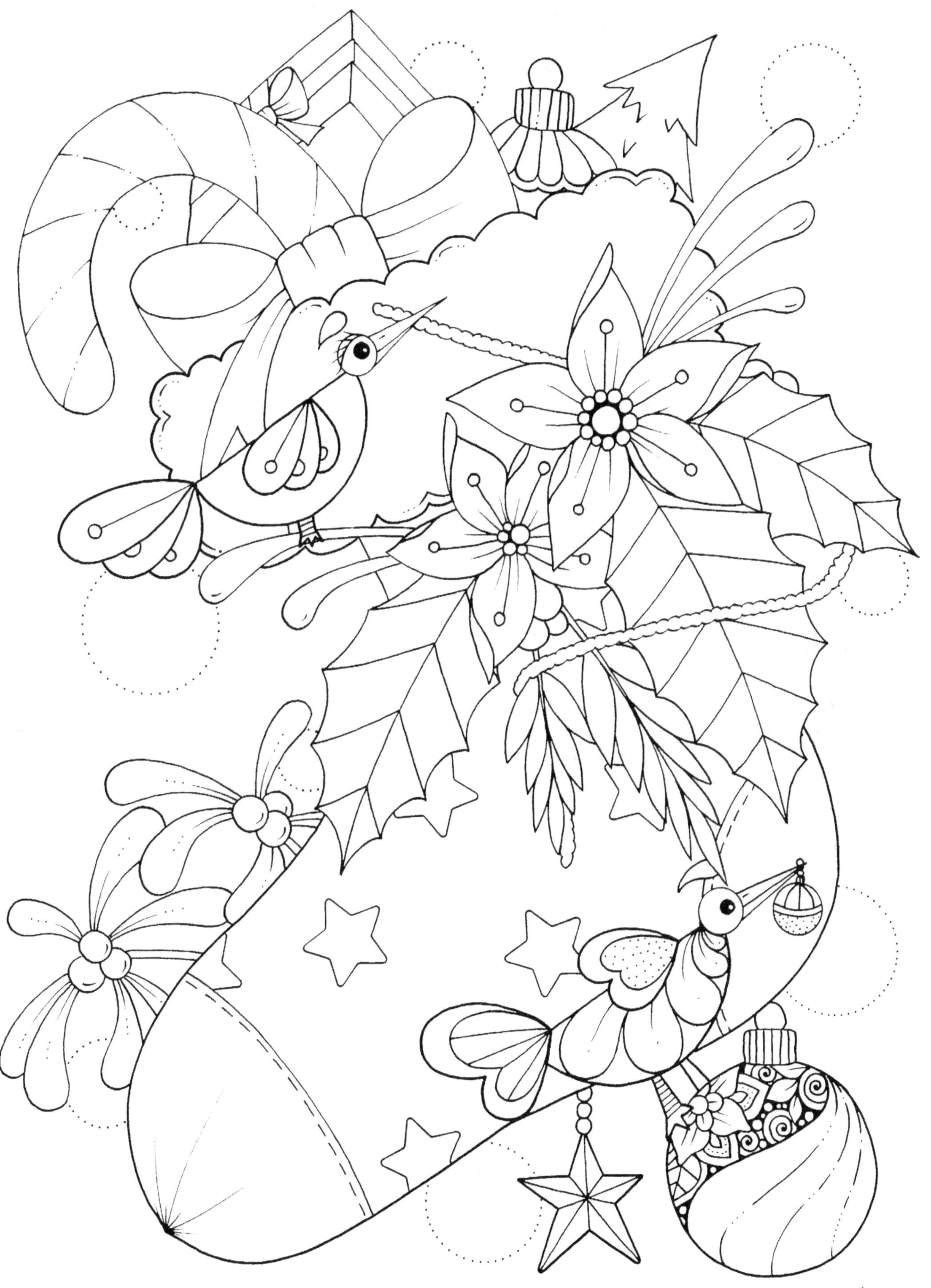

Colour Test Page

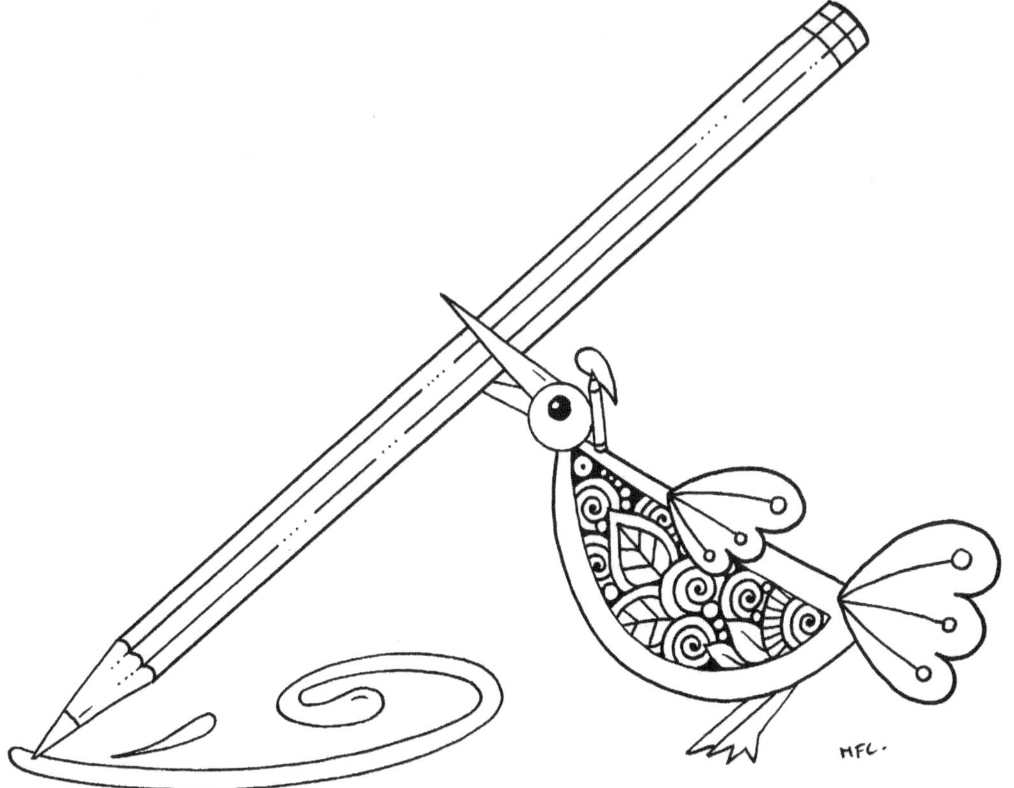

Colour Test Page

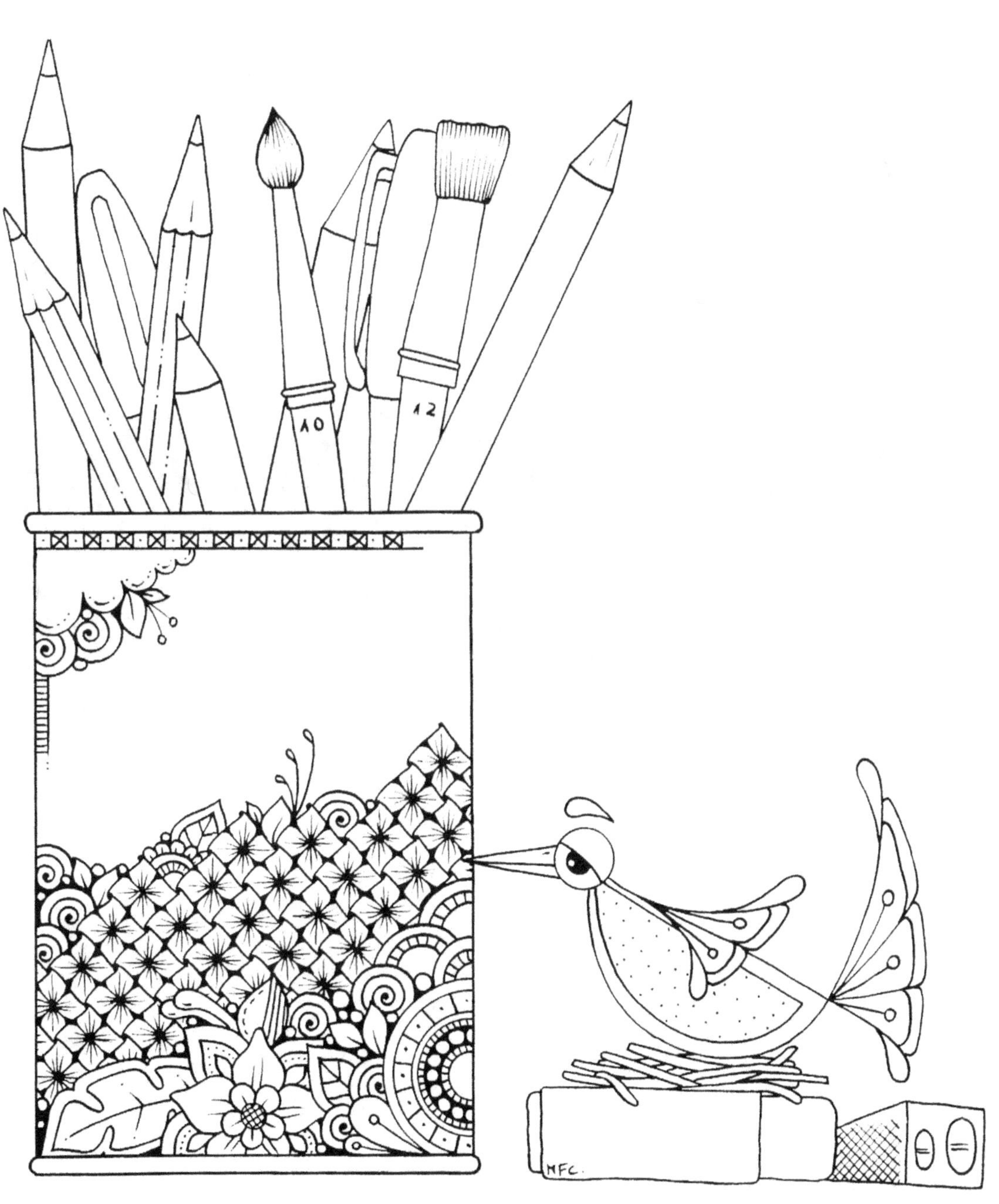

Colour Test Page

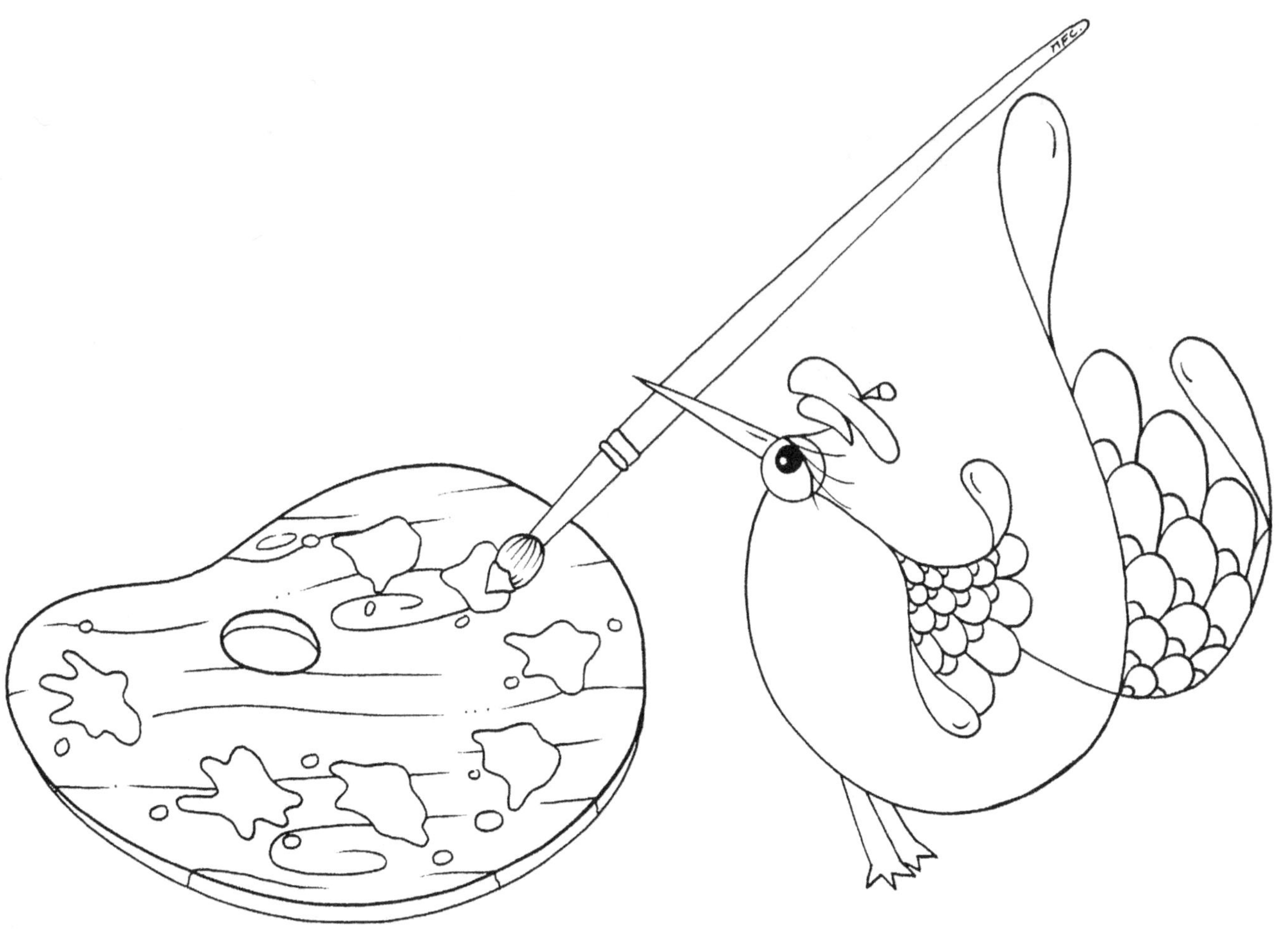

I will be really happy to see your colors and to share with you,
also join me on my Facebook page.
See you soon

https://www.facebook.com/MFC-Peinture-graphisme-illustrations